GW01184662

Naturally up to
160 calories
Everyday delicious treats!

It's sweet like regular cake, with real sugar, no artificial sweeteners, and only natural ingredients

The entire secret of how to bake delicious cakes with Greek yogurt and applesauce instead of oil

Naturally up to 160 calories. Everyday delicious treats!

ISBN-13 (pbk): 978-0-9855759-0-8
ISBN-13 (electronic): 978-0-9855759-1-5
Printed and bound in the United States of America 9 8 7 6 5 4 3 2 1

Trademarked names may appear in this book. Rather than use a trademark symbol with every occurrence of a trademarked name, we use the names only in an editorial fashion and to the benefit of the trademark owner, with no intention of infringement of the trademark.

May be purchased in bulk for academic, corporate, or promotional use.

eBook versions and licenses are also available.

For more information, please address Revital Federbush at revital.federbush@naturally-up-to.com

Library of Congress Control Number: 2012911845

For more information and questions: http://www.naturally-up-to.com

Designed by Aliza Ashkenazi Hayon
Photographs by Ronnie Federbush

This book is dedicated to my husband Ronnie and our two lovely daughters, Yahely and Daria - the real taste of my life

Acknowledgments

I literally could not have written this book without my family and friends.

I would especially like to thank my brother, Ram, for being the best taste tester around.

Special thanks to Chaim and Rachel Federbush—your help and kindness inspired me for all my life.

I also want to thank Susan and Jay Roth, Debbie and Jeff Schwartz, Jacob Cohen, Diane Fliegelman Cohen, Orly Gertner, Johnny Levin, and Amy Wasserman.

Finally, I would like to thank my father who taught me to love food.

I love you all.
Revital Federbush

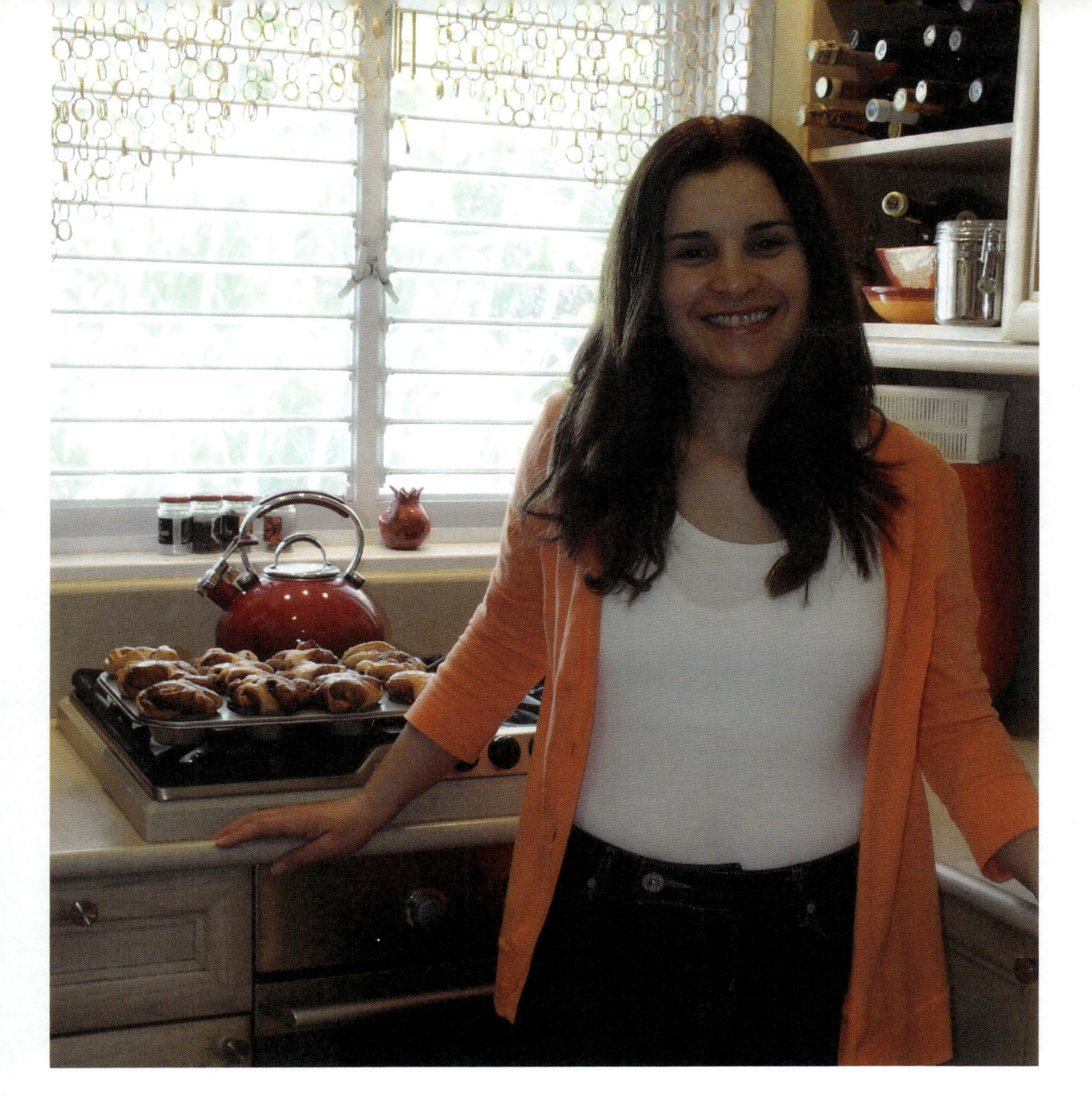

About the Author

Revital Federbush, forty-six, is a journalist covering health and nutrition issues for the last twenty-two years. She has over ten years of experience in developing recipes for cooking and baking.

The photos in this book are all original, with no use whatsoever of any imaging, photo-editing or alteration software.

Contents

Introduction

II just love cupcakes and muffins.

Well, doesn't everyone?

The problem is, I don't like being fat or going to the gym that much either. Now that's a bit of a conflict.

In this book I suggest a great solution to this conflict. You can eat a reasonably sized treat, the size of a standard muffin, every day without gaining weight. All of these treats are as sweet and as tasty as your ordinary desserts. Also, there is no use of artificial sweeteners or those "overly healthy" and strange substitutes like bran or carob powder. All of the ingredients are natural and healthy. And there's one more surprise: all of the recipes are only 120 to 160 calories per treat!

The recipes were inspired by my own personal diet pitfall. I always knew I'd be able to cope much better with my diet or with watching my weight if only I could have my "sweet half hour" a day. I love my four o'clock coffee break along with something sweet on the side. It just gives me the energy to get on with the rest of my day. Only I always wanted the real thing: a sweet, tasty cake. I didn't want to settle for energy bars crammed with artificial ingredients or for dietetic cakes made with artificial sweeteners that usually taste like cardboard. You just can't argue with the facts: when you have a real treat, you feel more satisfied because it really is tasty.

How do I cut down the calories? The facts are clear: the most fattening ingredient in a cake is the fat. One gram of fat is equal to nine calories. Compare that to carbohydrates (sugar, flour) at only about four calories per gram. Fat plays an important part in forming the texture of baked goods. It provides tenderness and moisture to cakes. After thousands of experiments I conducted in my kitchen, I came to the conclusion that if you use the correct ratios of healthy fat substitutes, such as Greek yogurt, applesauce, and orange juice, I can achieve similar results. The texture is soft and moist but with far fewer calories. A cup of oil is about 1,700 calories. A cup of applesauce is just 100 calories. A cup of 2 percent fat Greek yogurt is only 183 calories. That's where I cut down the calories.

In recent years, I deeply examined cake recipes. I discovered that there are recipes for delicious cakes that did not have much fat in them to begin with. There are many recipes for cakes that were never considered dietetic and contain very small amounts of fat and calories. Consider the famous Italian biscotti cookies. Italians love them, and so does the rest of the world. They are big and tasty, but they don't contain any fat and therefore, biscotti have relatively few calories. Without a doubt, I prefer these kinds of recipes to the recipes with two sticks of butter and 1,700 calories.

Here's another example: cupcakes with sweet and delicious meringue topping with a wonderful flavor reminiscent of a marshmallow candy. No one calls this a dietetic recipe, but this topping contains far fewer calories than, say, butter-based toppings. In fact, a cupcake with meringue icing contains less than a quarter of the calories! It's still deliciously sweet. I don't cut out the sugar; I just cut out the fat so it contains fewer calories and is also much healthier.

My goal in this book is to cut down the calories. I want to get the best deal I can get on the calories I use. The recipes in this book contain very little fat. For instance, instead of preparing the streusel muffins with massive amounts of butter, I just sprinkle the top of the muffins with a buttery crumb topping (streusel). The pastry gets a wonderful aroma and taste of butter at the very low cost of about thirty calories.

The same goes for the whipped cream: everyone agrees that whipped cream tastes wonderful. I dilute it with just the right amount of yogurt to significantly reduce the calories without compromising the unique flavor of whipped cream. This has even fooled children who love whipped cream. They couldn't tell the difference. In this way I avoid compromising on the real thing. The recipes in this book do not contain any substitute ingredients, such as artificial sweeteners or egg substitutes. I use only tasty, natural, and healthy ingredients. Now I can eat sweet cupcakes that are healthy and taste great without gaining weight.

The recipes in this book are an excellent solution for most dieters, even for overweight children. Many nutritionists now recommend that people not abstain entirely from the foods they love. Total abstinence often leads to uninhibited eating frenzies. It is okay to enjoy a daily treat that contains up to 10 percent of one's recommended calorie intake. The portions in this book are reasonably portioned and seeing as they contain up to only 160 calories, even children can enjoy a daily treat. All the recipes in this book have been tested on children as well as on adults. Only recipes that children liked were included in the book. While working on this book, I found an interesting phenomenon: when we get used to eating just one treat a day of sufficient size (for example, a standard-size muffin or two large cookies), the desire for sweets subsides. Suddenly, cakes and sweets become a part of life and are not as desirable. They become just like a lettuce leaf. No one craves a lettuce leaf in the middle of the day. This transformation does not occur in one day, but it does occur. Sweets become an integral part of life, like chicken or eggs or apples. This way you can maintain a balanced diet—both satisfying the need for sweets and controlling your weight throughout the years.

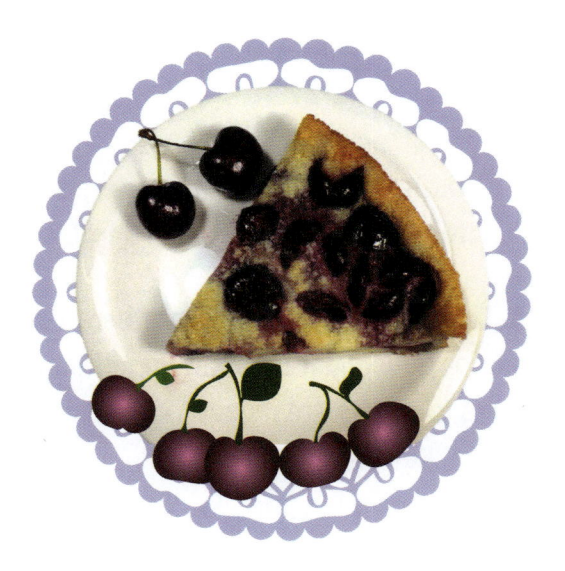

Frequently Asked Questions

The recipes in this book are not your usual recipes. Sometimes they call for slightly different techniques in order to reach maximum moisture and flavor.

Q: What happens if the recipe says fourteen treats but I got more?

A: Usually the amount of treats will be as stated in the recipe. Every recipe was tested numerous times. The amount of the batter is subject to slight changes, usually due to eggs. Very fresh eggs or eggs at room temperature will yield a better rising effect when whipped, hence producing more batter. Rarely is the difference due to the baking powder. For a single treat, the different volume could cause a difference of twenty calories or so, and therefore is not so substantial.

Q: My standard-size muffin pan has twelve cups. How do I bake a fourteen-muffin batch?

A: All treats are standard muffin size. Along with a standard twelve-cup muffin pan, you should get five to ten single-muffin tins. Just place the pan and the singles together on the oven rack.

Q: I usually either grease the pan or use paper liners. Why do the recipes call for placing paper liners in the pan and also greasing them?

A: The recipes are low fat, and there is nothing to prevent the treats from sticking to the pan or paper liner (another important role of fat). You should lightly grease the paper liners to get the treats out more easily.

Q: Why do some recipes call to further crush the applesauce in a blender?

A: Applesauce replaces the fat in the recipes. It should make the pastry moist and tender. Only when the applesauce is smooth enough will it do its job of adding moisture. If it is not smooth enough, you get a dry, at times brick-like, outcome. Pour the applesauce in a bowl. I usually use a stick blender. Any blender or food processor will do. It shouldn't take more than two minutes. Any unused applesauce can be frozen.

Q: Is it possible to save even more calories by replacing sugar with artificial sweetener?

A: Sugar has a role in pastries. Like fat, it also gives tenderness to the pastry. Sugar also gives the real, delicious taste of pastry to the cupcake. Therefore, substituting sugar with artificial sweetener might change the outcome completely.

Q: How do I measure the amounts—cups or ounces?

A: The most accurate way is to use scales. Usually the use of measuring cups and spoons is also very good. The only problem is that at times measuring tools are not accurate. It is, therefore, important to use a measurement tool from a known, reputable manufacturer. You can check if your measuring cups are accurate. Fill the measuring cup with water to the brim and weigh it. If the content of the cup is 240ml, the weight should be 240 grams. This will give you an indication of whether your measuring tools are accurate.

Q: The baking pan with water on the bottom of the oven—what is it for?

A: The water in the baking pan emits vapor that is needed in some of the recipes. It further improves the moistness of the treats.

Q: Should I use a regular or convection oven?

A: All recipes in this book are timed to be baked in regular ovens. Convection ovens work faster than regular ovens, as hot air moves more rapidly toward the cooler surface of the baked goods. This is why convection ovens require lower temperatures and shorter baking times. Take note that convection ovens could make slightly drier cakes.

Q: Can I skip the salt and make the cupcakes low sodium?

A: Yes, you can. Most people won't taste the difference.

Q: How many calories are in a cup of flour?

A: Information regarding calories per weight was taken directly from the packaging of the ingredients I used. These numbers are usually more accurate as they are based on lab results. I then weighed a standard cup of each ingredient to deduce the amount of calories per cup and other volume sizes. With this accurate information at hand, I added all the calories derived from each ingredient and divided by the number of servings. Please note that it is possible for this information to deviate by up to 5 percent. As we are dealing with so few calories, this is not that much of a problem. A cup of flour is about 433 calories.

Q: Can I change the recipes?

A: The balance between the liquid ingredients and the dry ingredients is critical to low-fat pastries. I would not recommend changing recipes at first. That being said, after you have gained some experience in preparing the recipes from this book, yes.

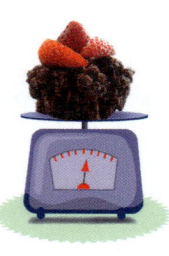

Q: What are the tools I need?

A: These are the tools you will need:

- Measuring cups and spoons. It is important to use precise measuring cups.
- Mixing bowls
- Standard muffin tin
- Individual muffin tins
- Paper liners
- Ice cream scoop. An ice cream scoop with a quick release mechanism is a convenient tool for filling muffin tins with batter. It is used to facilitate more uniform scoops to promote even baking.
- Wire rack—a tool for cooling baked goods quickly and evenly.
- Pastry bags. You can use either the disposable (easier to use) or the reusable (more environmentally friendly). For easy handling, choose a pastry bag that is between ten and fourteen inches long. The tips used to make the pastries shown in the pictures are the medium open star tip and the plain tip.

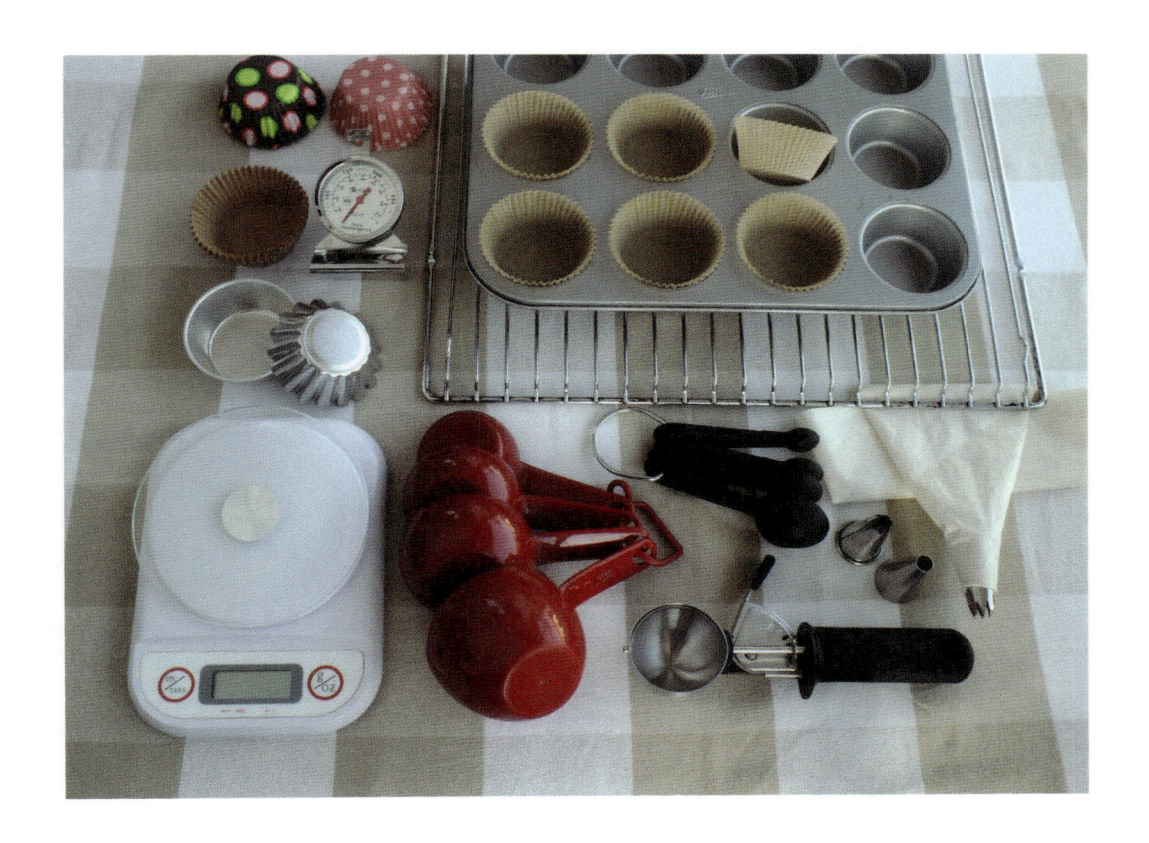

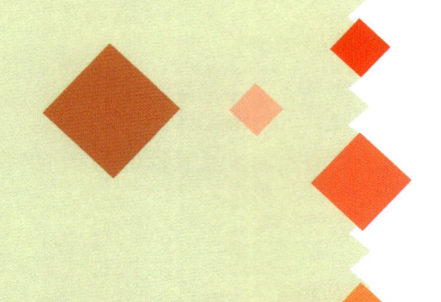

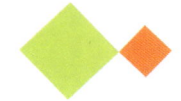

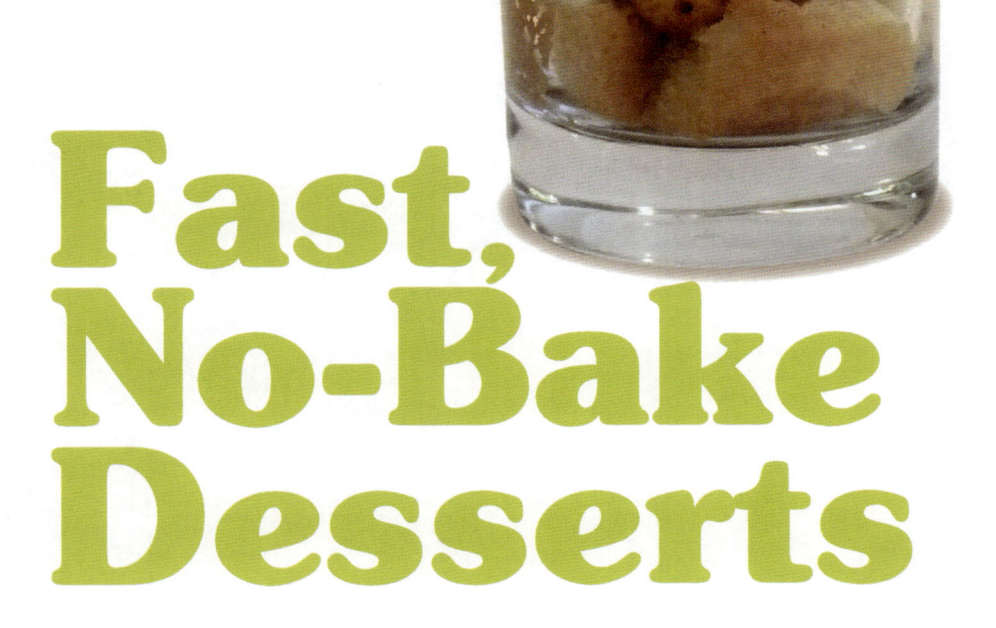

Fast, No-Bake Desserts

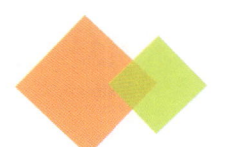

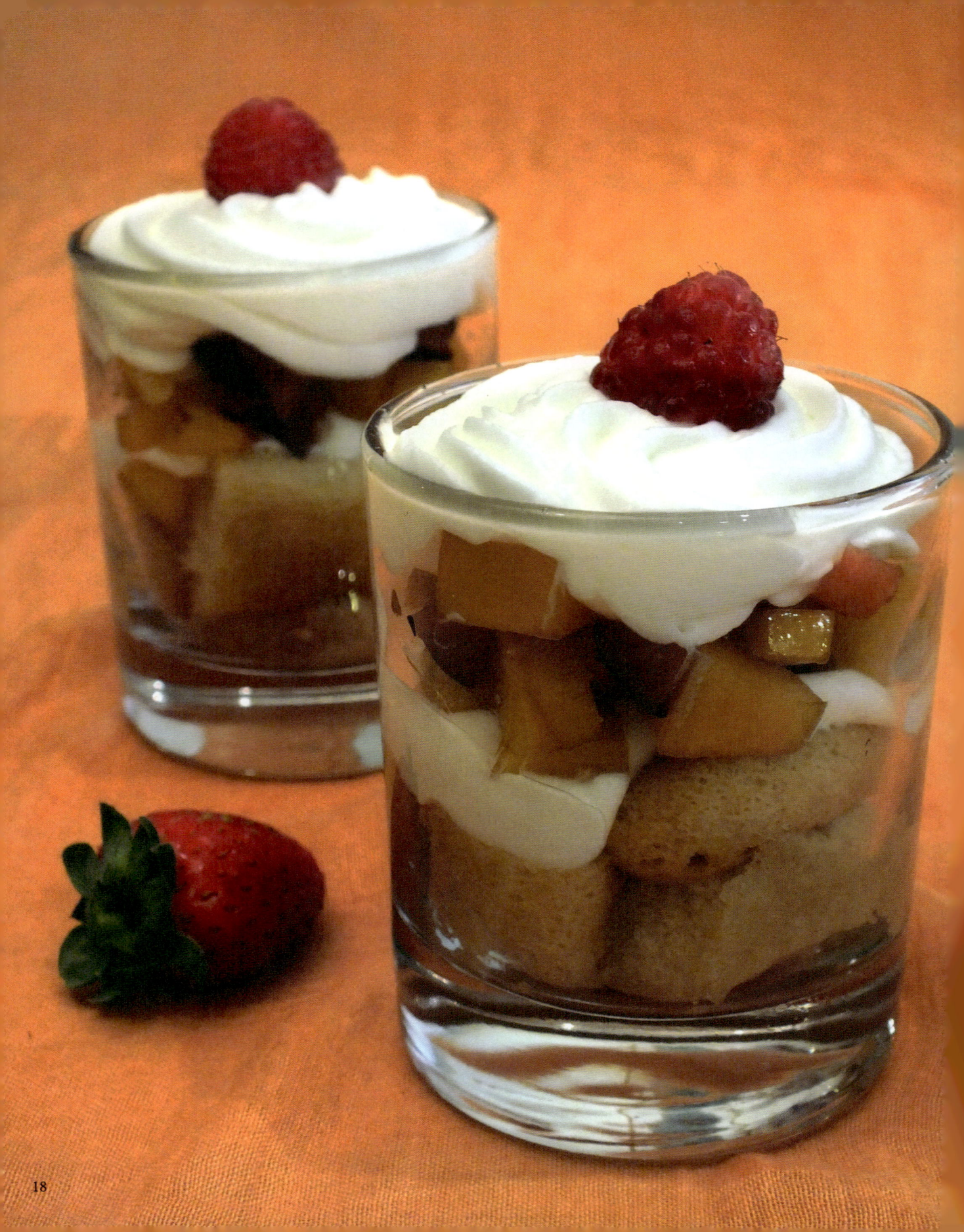

Trifle

Yield: 12 trifles | Per serving: 1 trifle – 154 calories

For the whipped cream:

1 cup heavy cream (double cream) 240 ml, 800 calories

¼ cup Greek yogurt 2%, 60 g, 45 calories

¼ cup milk (1% fat), 60 ml, 27 calories

1 tablespoon instant vanilla pudding, 10 g, 36 calories

4 tablespoons granulated sugar, 48 g, 180 calories

For the trifle:

18 ladyfingers (savoiardi in Italian), 150 g, 585 calories

½ cup orange juice, 120 ml, 54 calories

1½ cups fruit salad made from your favorite fresh fruit chopped into small pieces (blueberries, cherries, strawberries, peaches, and raspberries are all very nice), 210 g, 120 calories

Special equipment: Twelve 8-ounce (240 ml) dessert cups

In the bowl of an electric mixer, beat heavy cream, yogurt, milk, and instant pudding until soft peaks form. Sprinkle the sugar over cream, and beat until peaks return. Do not overbeat.

For each individual trifle, dip the ladyfingers in the orange juice for a second and cut in half. Lay three halves of ladyfingers in the bottom of each dessert cup, followed by fruit, then top with the whipped cream.
Cover each cup with plastic wrap and place in the refrigerator for at least four to six hours, preferably overnight, to allow the layers to blend.

Serve cold.
Trifles can be refrigerated up to two days in airtight containers.

Yogurt Pancakes

Yield: 16 3½-inch pancakes | Per serving: 2 pancakes plus 2 teaspoons maple syrup – 124 calories; 1 pancake – 45 calories; 1 teaspoon maple syrup – 17 calories

¾ cup all-purpose flour, 98 g, 325 calories

1 tablespoon granulated sugar, 12 g, 45 calories

1 teaspoon baking powder

½ teaspoon fine salt

1 cup Greek yogurt 2%, 240 g, 180 calories

2 extra-large eggs, 160 calories

½ cup water

1 teaspoon vanilla extract, 4 g, 12 calories

Mix the dry ingredients together in a large bowl. Whisk the yogurt, eggs, water, and vanilla together in another bowl. Add the wet ingredients to the dry ingredients, whisking just enough to combine.

Heat up a nonstick pan over medium-high heat, and spray with nonstick baking spray. Using an ice cream scoop or a small ladle, pour about ¼ cup (60 ml) of pancake batter onto the hot pan, spacing the pancakes a few inches apart. If the batter is too thick, add 1 to 3 tablespoons of water. When the bottoms of the pancakes are brown and bubbles start to appear on the top surfaces of the pancakes, turn over. Cook until lightly browned. Repeat with remaining batter.

Serve immediately.

Chocolate Cornflakes Crispy Treats
Yield: 12 treats | Per serving: 1 treat – 127 calories

4 cups cornflakes, 112 g, 400 calories

8 ounces semi-sweet chocolate, cut into ½-inch chunks (or 1⅓ cups chocolate chips), 224 g, 1,120 calories

¼ cup plus 1 tablespoon of water

Line standard muffin tin with baking cups and spray with nonstick spray.

Put the cornflakes in a large mixing bowl.
Melt the chocolate with the water in a small pan over low heat and mix thoroughly until the chocolate is melted and the mixture is combined and smooth. Remove from heat and let cool for approximately five minutes. Pour chocolate mixture over cornflakes. Mix together quickly and distribute evenly with two spoons among the baking cups. Cover the tin loosely with a plastic bag and freeze for at least one hour.

Box them up and keep in the refrigerator for a few days.

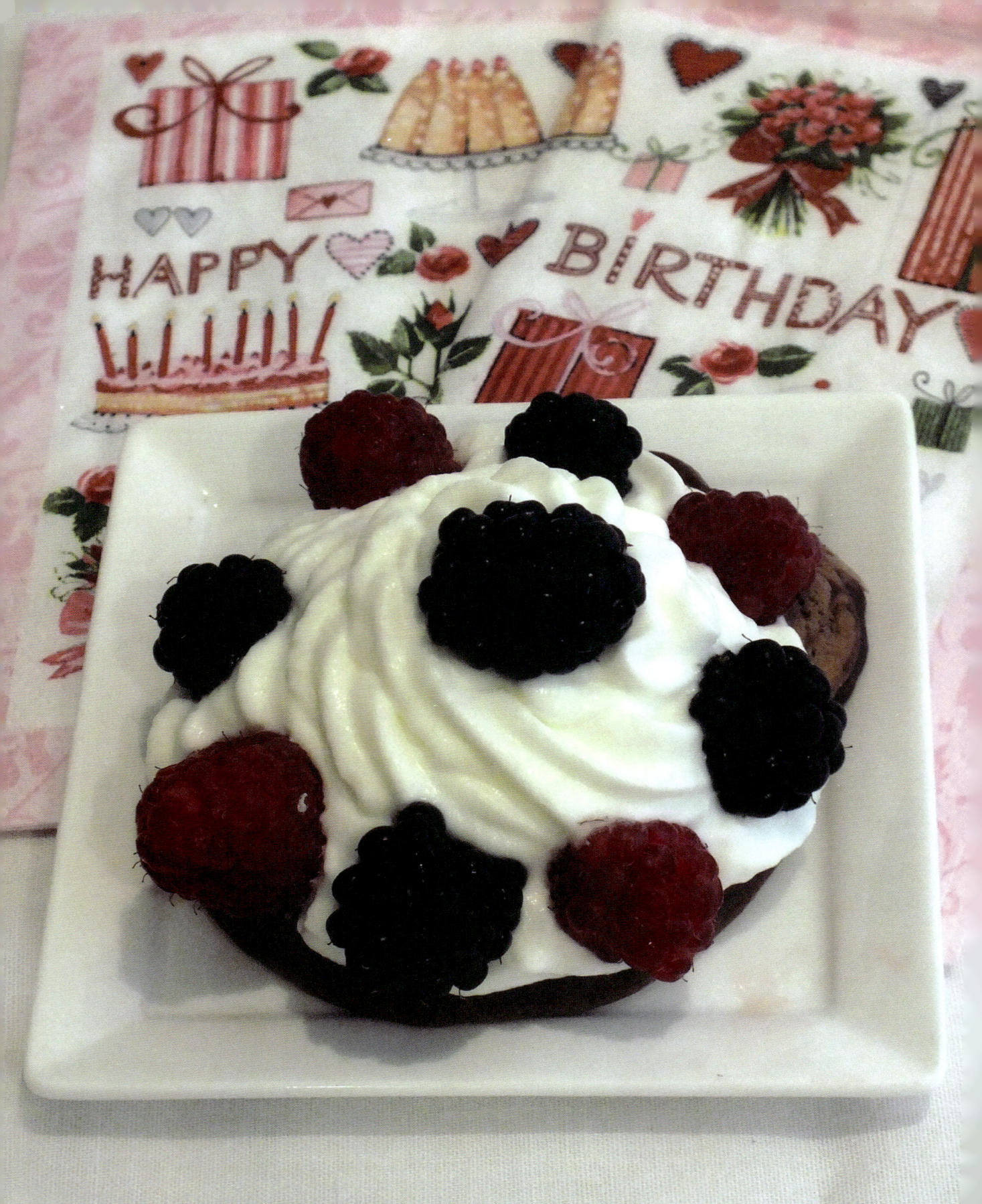

Special Birthday Treats
Yield: 12 treats | Per serving: 1 treat – 130 calories

For the pancakes:

⅔ cup all-purpose flour, 86 g, 286 calories

2 teaspoons granulated sugar, 8 g, 30 calories

1 teaspoon baking powder

Pinch fine salt

2 extra-large eggs, 160 calories

⅓ cup low-fat buttermilk, 82 g, 33 calories

¼ cup milk (1% fat), 60 ml, 27 calories

For the fruit mixture:

1½ cups fruit salad made from your favorite fresh fruit chopped into bite-sized pieces (blueberries, cherries, strawberries, peaches, and raspberries are all very nice), 210 g, 120 calories

3 tablespoons orange juice, 45 ml, 20 calories

1½ tablespoons powdered (confectioners') sugar, 12 g, 48 calories

For the whipped cream:

¾ cup heavy cream (double cream), 180 ml, 600 calories

¼ cup Greek yogurt 2%, 60 g, 45 calories

¼ cup milk (1% fat), 60 ml, 27 calories

1 tablespoon instant vanilla pudding, 10 g, 36 calories

3 tablespoons granulated sugar, 36 g, 135 calories

Pancakes:

Mix the dry ingredients together in a large bowl. Whisk the eggs, buttermilk, and milk together in another bowl. Add the wet ingredients to the dry ingredients, whisking just enough to combine.

Heat up a nonstick pan over medium-high heat, and spray with nonstick baking spray. Using an ice cream scoop or a small ladle, pour about ¼ cup (60 ml) of pancake batter onto the hot pan, spacing the pancakes a few inches apart. When the bottoms of the pancakes are brown and bubbles start to appear on the top surfaces of the pancakes, turn over. Cook until lightly browned. Repeat with remaining batter. Put the twelve pancakes on the side.

Fruit mixture:

Combine the fruits with the orange juice and the powdered sugar.

Whipped Cream:

In bowl of an electric mixer, beat heavy cream, yogurt, milk, and instant pudding until soft peaks form. Sprinkle the sugar over cream, and beat until peaks return. Do not overbeat.

Assemble (just before serving):

For each individual treat, place one pancake on small plate. Pour a little bit of fruit syrup from the fruit salad over the pancakes and then evenly distribute the fruit on top of the pancakes. To finish, fill a pastry bag fitted with a medium star tip with whipped cream and pipe onto each pancake.

Serve immediately.

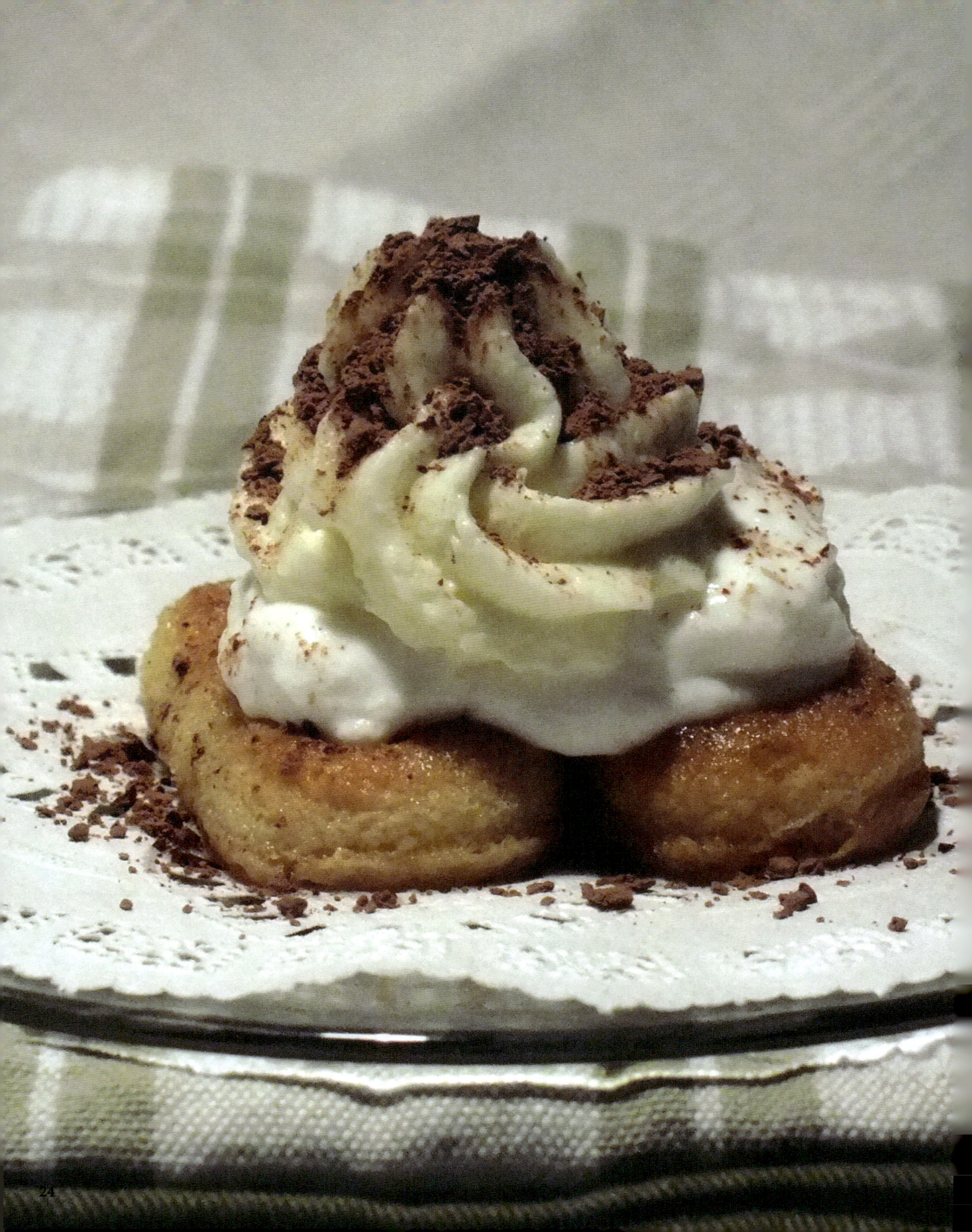

Tiramisu

Yield: 12 Tiramisus | Per serving: 1 Tiramisu – 147 calories

For the yogurt mixture:

¾ cup Greek yogurt 2%, 180 g,
135 calories

4 tablespoons granulated sugar, 48 g,
180 calories

1 teaspoon vanilla extract, 4 g,
12 calories

For the whipped cream:

¾ cup heavy cream (double cream)
180 ml, 600 calories

¼ cup Greek yogurt 2%, 60 g,
45 calories

¼ cup milk (1% fat), 60 ml,
27 calories

1 tablespoon instant vanilla pudding,
10 g, 36 calories

3 tablespoons granulated sugar, 36 g,
135 calories

1 cup espresso or strong coffee at
room temperature

18 ladyfingers (savoiardi in Italian),
150 g, 585 calories

1 tablespoon cocoa powder, 5 g,
10 calories

Special equipment: Twelve 8-ounce (240 ml) dessert cups

Yogurt mixture:
In a small bowl, whisk the yogurt, 4 tablespoons sugar, and vanilla until the mixture is combined and smooth. Set aside.

Whipped cream:
In bowl of an electric mixer, beat heavy cream, yogurt, milk, and instant pudding until soft peaks form. Sprinkle the sugar over cream and beat until peaks return. Do not overbeat.

Place the coffee in a medium shallow bowl.
For each individual Tiramisu, dip the ladyfingers in the coffee for a second and cut in half. Lay three halves of ladyfingers in the bottom of each cup, followed by a spoon of yogurt, then the whipped cream.
Cover each bowl with plastic wrap and place in the refrigerator for at least four to six hours, preferably overnight, to allow the layers to blend.
Serve cold.
Just before serving, dust with cocoa powder.
Tiramisu can be refrigerated up to two days in airtight containers.

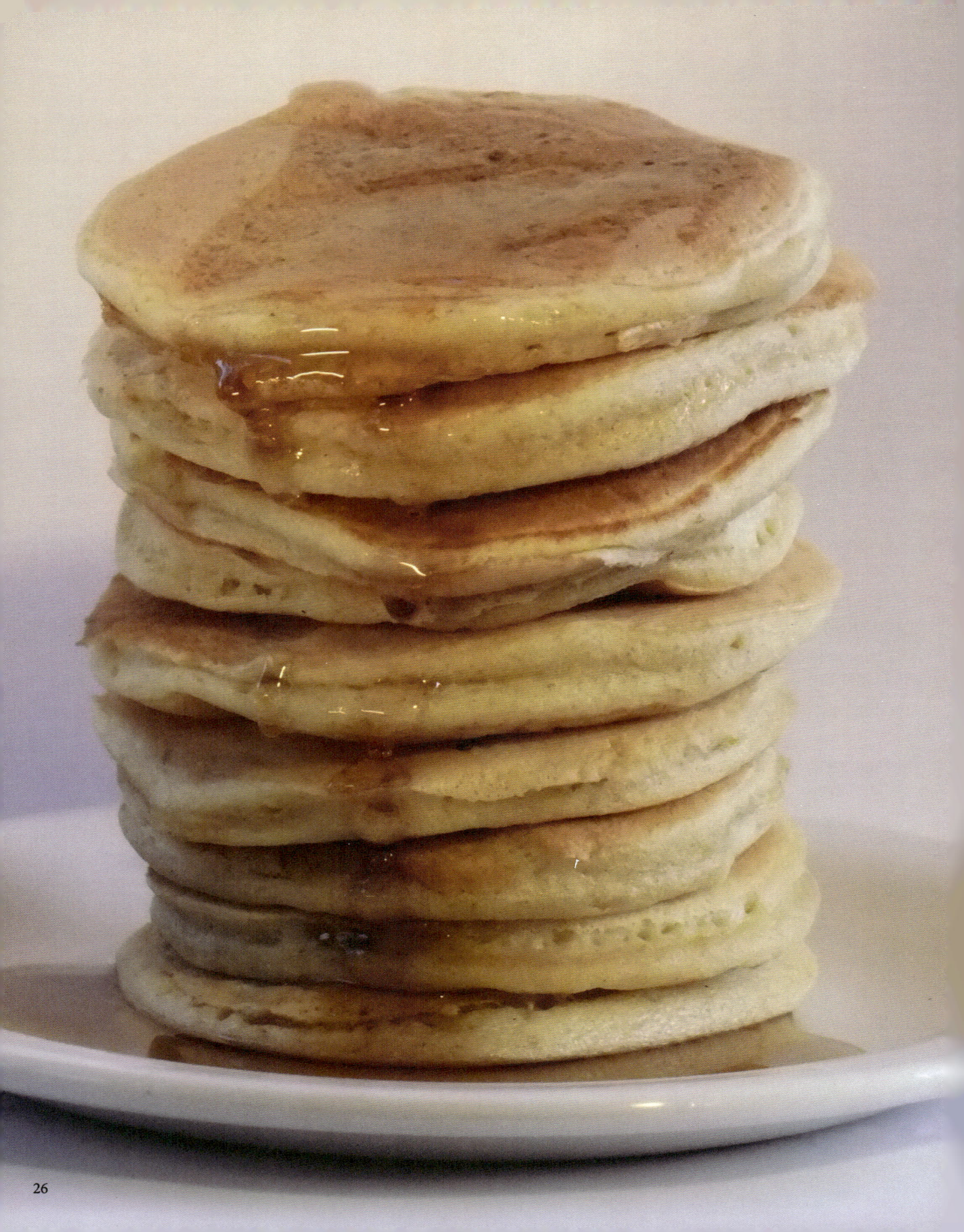

Whipped Pancakes

Yield: 36 3½-inch pancake | Per serving: 3 pancakes plus 3 teaspoons of maple syrup – 159 calories; 1 pancake – 36 calories; 1 teaspoon maple syrup – 17 calories

3 extra-large eggs, separated, 240 calories

½ teaspoon fine salt

2 tablespoons granulated sugar, 24 g, 90 calories

2 cups all-purpose flour, 260 g, 866 calories

1 cup low-fat buttermilk, 245 g, 98 calories

1 teaspoon vanilla extract, 4 g, 12 calories

2 cups water

2½ teaspoons baking powder

With an electric mixer—the bowl and beaters must be clean and free of grease—beat the egg whites and the salt on low-medium speed until foamy, about one minute. Add the sugar and continue to beat, but not too much (about two minutes). Transfer the egg whites to a medium bowl and put aside.

In the same mixer bowl (no need to wash), mix the flour, egg yolks, buttermilk, vanilla and water until incorporated. Sift the baking powder and combine.
Using a rubber spatula or a whisk, fold a small amount of egg whites into the flour mixture to lighten the batter. Add the remaining egg whites, folding until incorporated (small lumps are okay).

Heat up a nonstick pan over medium-high heat, and spray with nonstick baking spray. Using an ice cream scoop or a small ladle, pour about ¼ cup (60 ml) of pancake batter onto the hot pan, spacing the pancakes a few inches apart. When the bottoms of the pancakes are brown and bubbles start to appear on the top surfaces of the pancakes, turn over. Cook until lightly browned. Repeat with remaining batter.
Serve immediately.

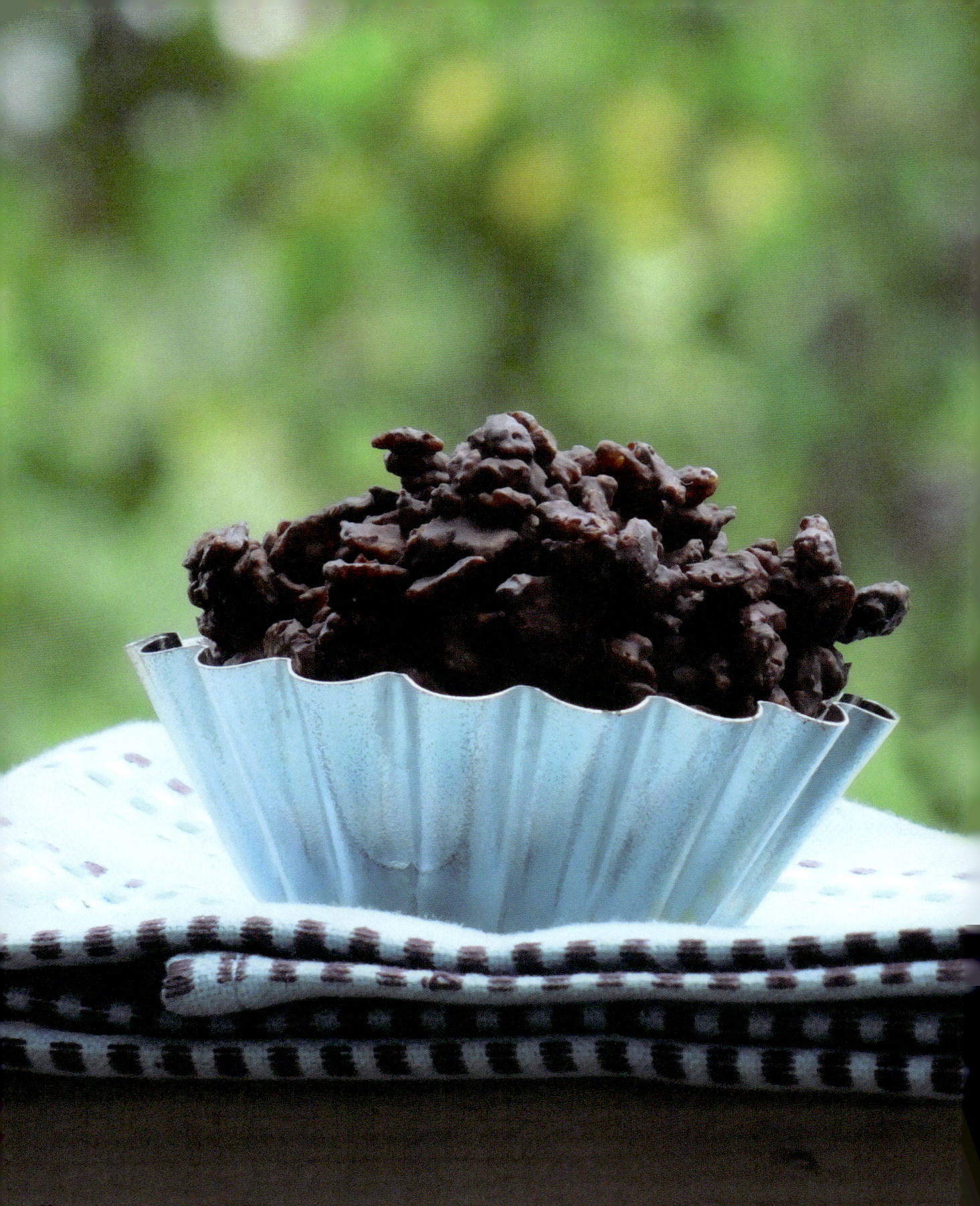

Chocolate Rice Krispies Treats
Yield: 12 treats | Per serving: 1 treat – 138 calories

3¾ cups Rice Krispies, 100 g, 390 calories

¼ cup plus 1 tablespoon of water

9 ounces semi-sweet chocolate, cut into ½-inch chunks (or 1½ cups chocolate chips), 252 g, 1,260 calories

Line standard muffin tin with baking cups and spray with nonstick spray.

Put the Rice Krispies in a large mixing bowl.
Add water to chocolate in a small saucepan over very low heat, and stir until chocolate is melted and mixture is completely smooth. Remove from heat and let cool approximately five minutes. Pour into Rice Krispies and mix together quickly. Using two spoons, distribute into baking cups. Press down gently on each. Cover the tin loosely with a plastic bag and freeze at least one hour.

Box them up and keep in the refrigerator for a few days.

Chocolate

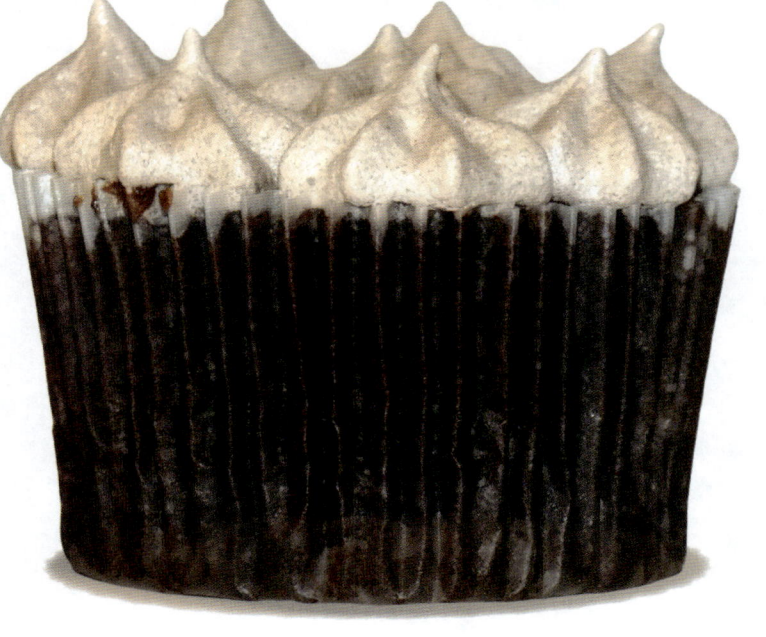

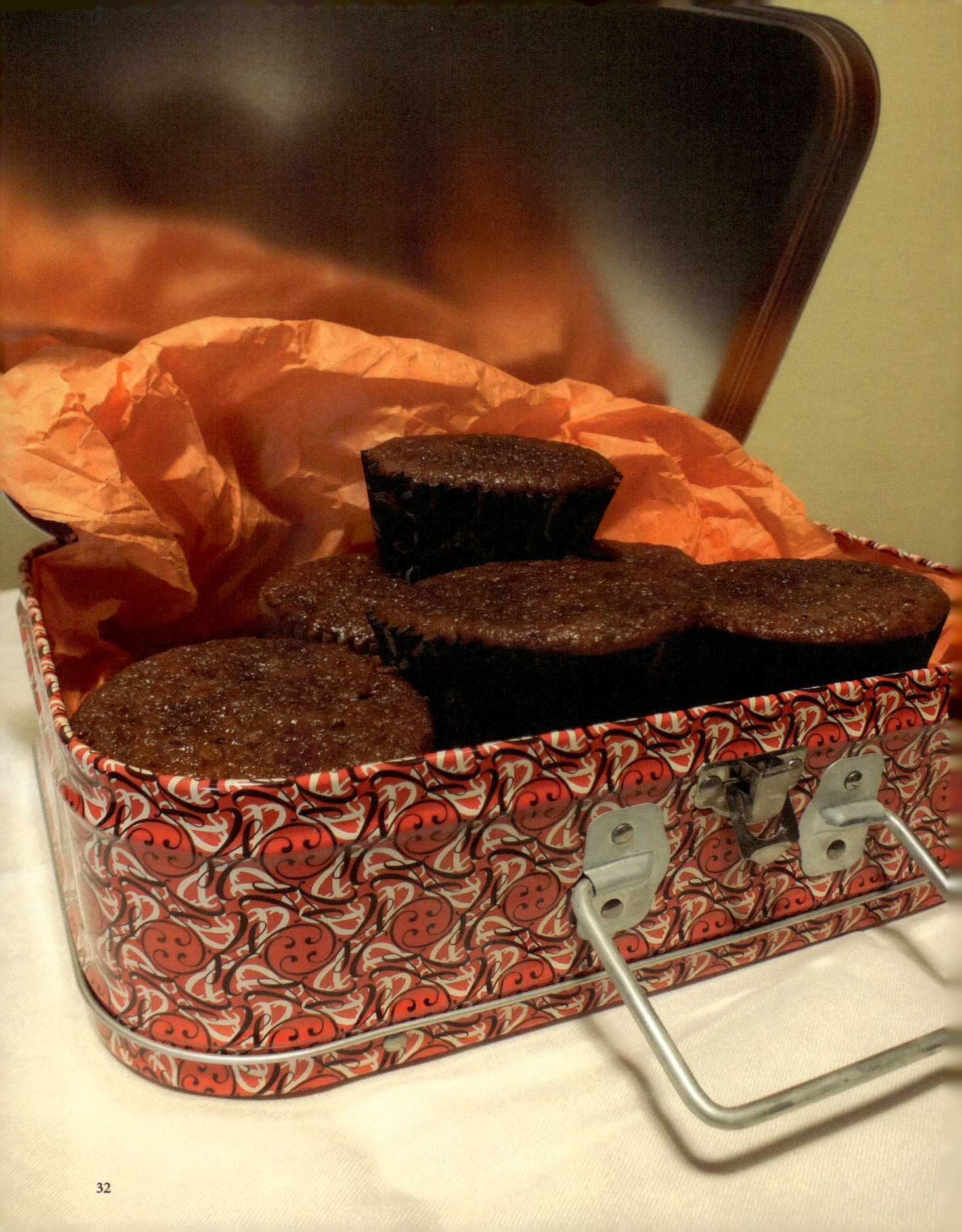

Chocolate-Orange Muffins
Yield: 15 muffins | Per serving: 1 muffin - 149 calories

3 tablespoons of water

2½ ounce (5 tablespoons) semi-sweet chocolate chips, 70 g, 350 calories

1½ cups all-purpose flour, 195 g, 650 calories

1½ teaspoons baking powder

½ teaspoon baking soda

1 cup granulated sugar, 200 g, 750 calories

1 cup minus 1 tablespoon Greek yogurt 2%, 225 g, 170 calories

1/2 cup orange juice, 180 ml, 81 calories

3 extra-large eggs, 240 calories

¼ teaspoon fine salt

Preheat oven to 340°F (170°C).
Line standard muffin tin with baking cups, and spray with nonstick spray.
Put a pan (or any similar baking dish) with 1 cup of water on the bottom rack of the oven.

Add water to chocolate in a small saucepan over very low heat, and stir until chocolate is melted and mixture is completely smooth. Remove from heat and let cool approximately five minutes.
Sift the flour, baking powder, and baking soda into a large bowl. Mix in the sugar.
In a medium-sized bowl, whisk the Greek yogurt, orange juice, and the chocolate mixture. Stir until the mixture is combined and smooth.

With an electric mixer, with the whisk attachment, beat the whole eggs together with salt on high speed until they are thick and fluffy (about two minutes).
Gently fold the yogurt mixture into the eggs until incorporated.
Make a well in the flour mixture, pour in the liquid mixture, and stir just to combine (do not over-mix or you will have tough muffins).
Use an ice cream scoop to distribute the batter evenly among the baking cups, filling each 90 percent full.
Bake for approximately twenty-five to thirty minutes or until a toothpick tests clean or with few crumbs. Cool in the pan for a few minutes before removing to a cooling rack.
Muffins can be stored up to two days in the refrigerator in airtight containers.

Chocolate-Banana Cupcakes

Yield: 15 cupcakes | Per serving: 1 cupcake - 152 calories

For the cupcakes:

5 tablespoons of water

4 ounces semi-sweet chocolate, cut into ½-inch chunks (or ⅔ cup chocolate chips), 112 g, 560 calories

¾ cup all-purpose flour, 98 g, 325 calories

1 tablespoon cocoa powder, 5 g, 10 calories

¾ teaspoon baking powder

¾ teaspoon baking soda

½ cup granulated sugar, 100 g, 375 calories

¾ cup ripe bananas (approximately 1½ large bananas), 160 g, 142 calories

¾ cup Greek yogurt 2%, 180 g, 135 calories

1 teaspoon vanilla extract, 4 g, 12 calories

¼ cup milk (1% fat), 60 ml, 27 calories

1 extra-large egg, 80 calories

3 extra-large egg yolks, 192 calories

¼ teaspoon fine salt

For the meringue:

2 egg whites at room temperature, 32 calories

¼ teaspoon fine salt

½ cup granulated sugar, 100 g, 375 calories

1 tablespoon cocoa powder, 5 g, 10 calories

Preheat oven to 340°F (170°C).

Line a standard muffin tin with paper liners (or baking cups), and spray with nonstick baking spray.
Put a pan (or any similar baking dish) with 1 cup of water on the bottom rack of the oven.
Add water to chocolate in a small saucepan over very low heat, and stir until chocolate is melted and mixture is completely smooth. Remove from heat and let cool approximately five minutes.
Sift the flour, cocoa, baking powder, and baking soda together in a large mixing bowl. Mix in the sugar.
Puree the bananas in a blender or a food processor (the bananas need to be finely pureed and smooth) and then measure ¾ cup.

In a medium bowl, whisk together the yogurt, vanilla, bananas, milk, and chocolate mixture. Stir until the mixture is combined and smooth.
With an electric mixer, with the whisk attachment beat the whole egg, 3 egg yolks, and the salt on high speed until the batter is thick and fluffy (about two minutes).
Gently fold the yogurt-chocolate mixture into the eggs until incorporated.
Make a well in the flour mixture and pour in the liquid mixture. Stir just to combine (don't over-mix or you will have tough cupcakes).
Use an ice cream scoop to distribute the batter evenly among the baking cups, filling each 90 percent full. Bake for approximately twenty-five minutes, until firm but not fully baked.

Make the meringue when the cupcakes are in the oven:
With an electric mixer—the bowl and beaters must be clean and free of grease—beat the egg whites on low-medium speed until foamy. Add the salt and continue to beat until they hold soft peaks. Add the sugar, a little at a time, and continue to beat until the meringue holds very stiff peaks. Sift cocoa over the egg whites and gently fold in until just blended. Transfer meringue to a pastry bag fitted with a small open-star tip.

Remove the cupcakes from the oven and pipe five to seven starbursts around perimeter of the warm cupcakes, then pipe another starburst in the center. Return to the oven and bake about three to five minutes. Don't over-bake or you will have dry cupcakes.
Cool in the pan for a few minutes before removing to a cooling rack.
Cupcakes can be refrigerated up to two days in airtight containers.

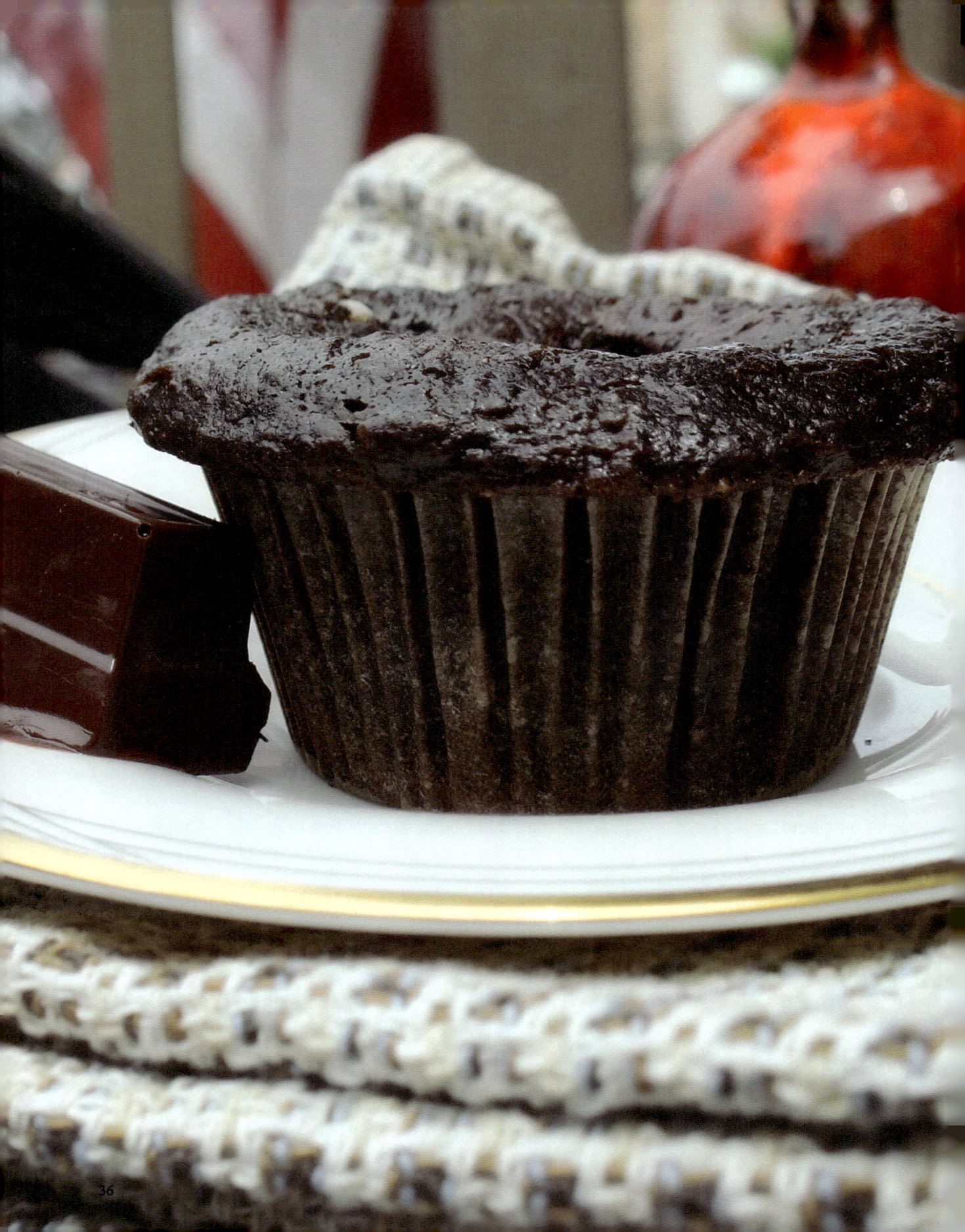

Fudgy Chocolate Treats

Yield: 13 treats | Per serving: 1 treat - 145 calories

6 tablespoons of water

5½ ounces semi-sweet chocolate, cut into ½-inch chunks, 154 g, 770 calories

¾ cup all-purpose flour, 98 g, 325 calories

1 tablespoon cocoa powder, 5 g, 10 calories

¾ teaspoon baking powder

¾ teaspoon baking soda

½ cup granulated sugar, 100 g, 375 calories

½ cup unsweetened applesauce, 105 g, 43 calories

¾ cup Greek yogurt 2%, 180 g, 135 calories

1 teaspoon vanilla extract, 4 g, 12 calories

½ cup milk (1% fat), 120 ml, 54 calories

2 extra-large eggs, 160 calories

½ teaspoon fine salt

Preheat oven to 340°F (170°C).

Line a standard muffin tin with paper liners (or baking cups), and spray with nonstick baking spray.

Put a pan (or any similar baking dish) with 1 cup of water on the bottom rack of the oven.

Add water to chocolate in a small saucepan over very low heat, and stir until chocolate is melted and mixture is completely smooth. Remove from heat and let cool approximately five minutes.

Sift the flour, cocoa, baking powder, and baking soda together in a large mixing bowl. Mix in the sugar.

Puree the applesauce in a blender or a food processor (the applesauce needs to be finely pureed and smooth) and then measure ½ cup.

In a medium bowl, whisk together the applesauce, yogurt, vanilla, milk, and chocolate mixture. Stir until the mixture is combined and smooth.

With an electric mixer, with the whisk attachment, beat the whole eggs and the salt on high speed until the batter is thick and fluffy (about two minutes).

Gently fold the yogurt-chocolate mixture into the eggs until incorporated.

Make a well in the flour mixture and pour in the liquid mixture. Stir just to combine (do not over-mix or you will have tough cakes).

Use an ice cream scoop to distribute the batter evenly among the baking cups, filling each 90 percent full. Bake for approximately thirty minutes (do not over-bake or you will have dry cakes). Cool in the pan for a few minutes before removing to a cooling rack.

Cakes can be stored up to two days in the refrigerator.

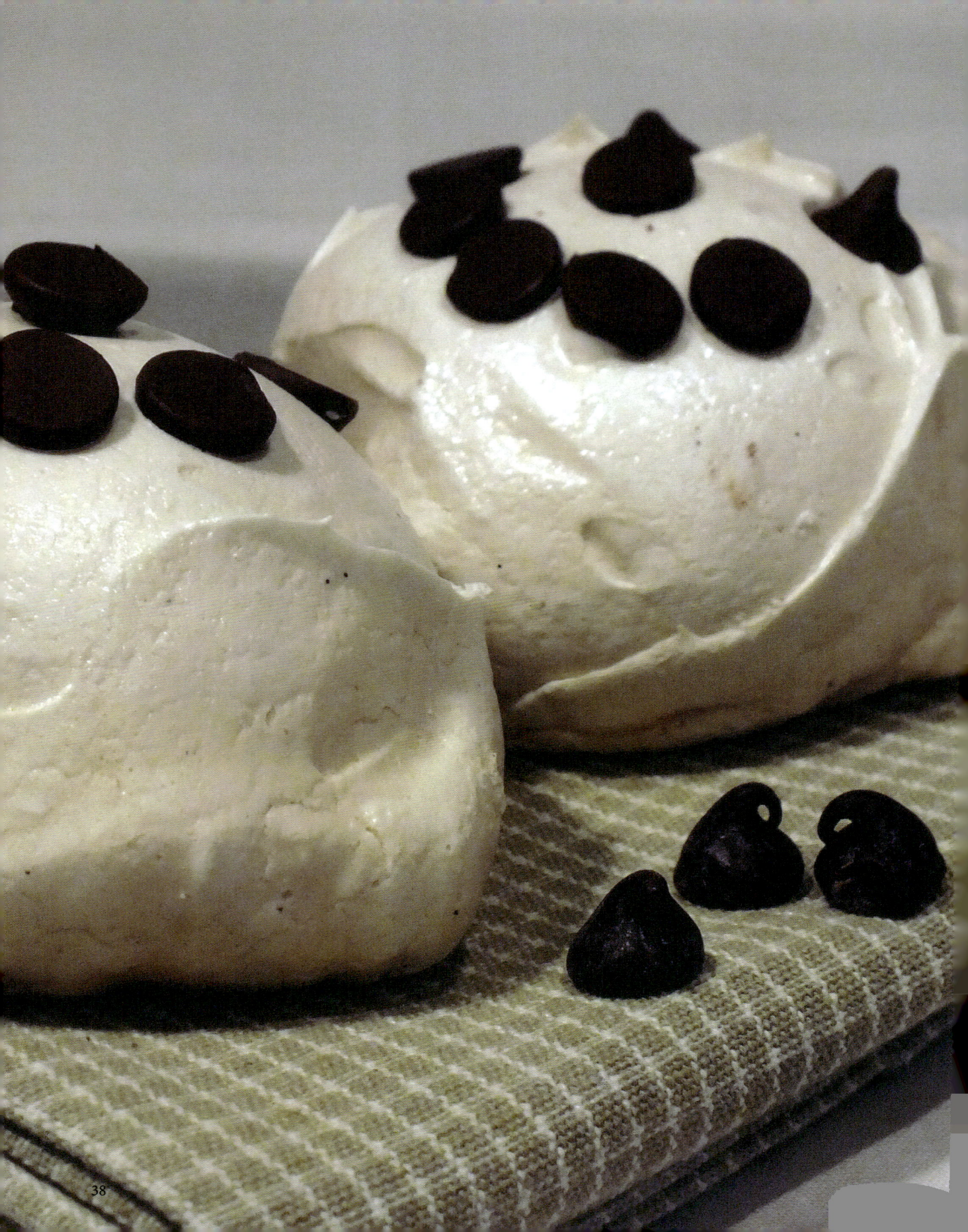

Chocolate Chip Meringue Cookies

Yield: 12 extra large cookies | Per serving: 2 cookies - 142 calories; 1 cookie - 71 calories

2 extra-large egg whites, 32 calories

¼ teaspoon fine salt

½ teaspoon white vinegar

¾ cup granulated sugar, 150 g, 562 calories

1 teaspoon vanilla extract, 4 g, 12 calories

1 tablespoon cornstarch (corn flour), 8 g, 30 calories

1½ ounce (¼ cup) semi-sweet chocolate chips, 42 g, 210 calories

Preheat the oven to 230°F (110°C).
Line a baking sheet with parchment paper.

Combine egg whites, salt, and white vinegar together in the bowl of an electric mixer—the bowl and beaters must be clean and free of grease— and beat on high speed until soft peaks form (about four minutes). Add the sugar, a little at a time, and continue to beat until the egg whites holds very stiff peaks. Beat in the vanilla extract. Sift in the cornstarch and fold with a rubber spatula.
Use an ice cream scoop or two spoons to spoon mounds of meringue onto the prepared sheets. Sprinkle the top of the cookies evenly with the chocolate chips.

Bake for about two hours, rotating the baking sheet from front to back to ensure even baking. The meringues are done when they are pale in color and fairly crisp. Turn off the heat and cool the meringues in the oven for an hour, propping the door open with a wooden spoon.
The cookies can be covered and stored up to two days at room temperature in airtight containers.

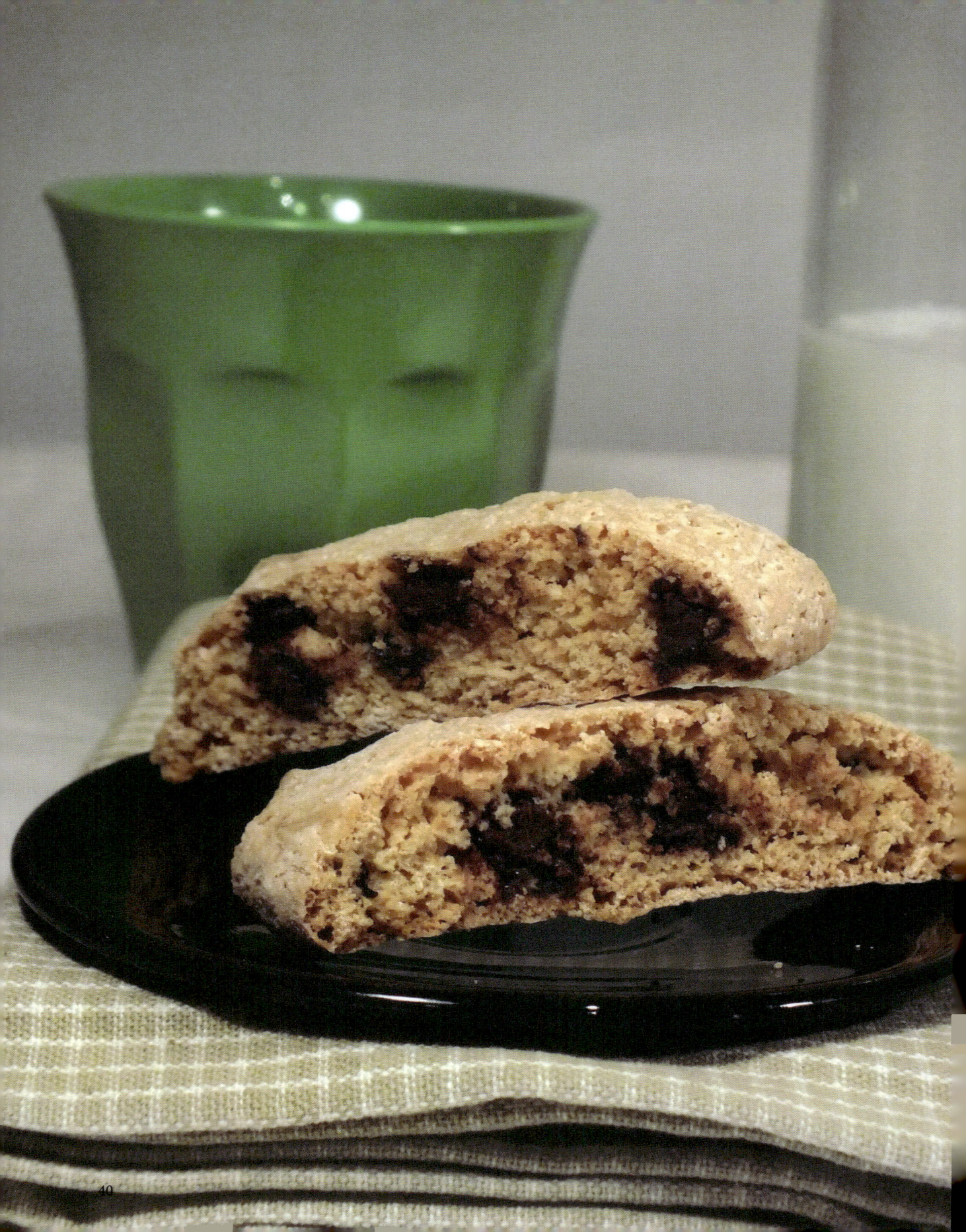

Chocolate Chip Biscotti

Yield: 40 biscotti | Per serving: 2 biscotti - 140 calories; 1 biscotto - 70 calories

2½ cups all-purpose flour, 325 g, 1,083 calories

2 teaspoons baking powder

1 teaspoon ground cinnamon, 2 g, 6 calories

1 cup granulated sugar, 200 g, 750 calories

¼ teaspoon salt

3 extra-large eggs, 240 calories

1 teaspoon vanilla extract, 4 g, 12 calories

5 ounces (¾ cup plus 1 tablespoon) semi-sweet chocolate chips, 140 g, 700 calories

Preheat oven to 350°F (175°C).

Line a baking sheet with parchment paper.

In the bowl of an electric mixer, combine the flour, baking powder, cinnamon, sugar, and salt. In another small bowl, whisk the eggs and the vanilla. Gradually add the egg mixture to the flour mixture and beat until a dough forms. If the dough does not form, add one to three tablespoons of water. Combine the chocolate chips.

With floured hands (the dough is quite sticky), divide the dough into two pieces. On a lightly floured surface, roll each half of dough into a log about sixteen inches (forty centimeters) long and two inches (five centimeters) wide. Transfer the logs to the prepared baking sheet, spacing about four inches (ten centimeters) apart. Logs will spread during baking. Bake until firm to the touch, about twenty-five to thirty minutes. Let cool for about twenty minutes.

Reduce oven temperature to 300°F (150°C).

Cut the logs into slices about ½-inch (1¼ cm) thick using a serrated knife; cut each log into twenty pieces. Arrange the slices, cut side down, on the baking sheet. Bake ten minutes then turn slices over and bake another ten minutes, or until golden brown. Remove from oven and let cool on a wire rack.

Cookies can be stored in an airtight container for a month.

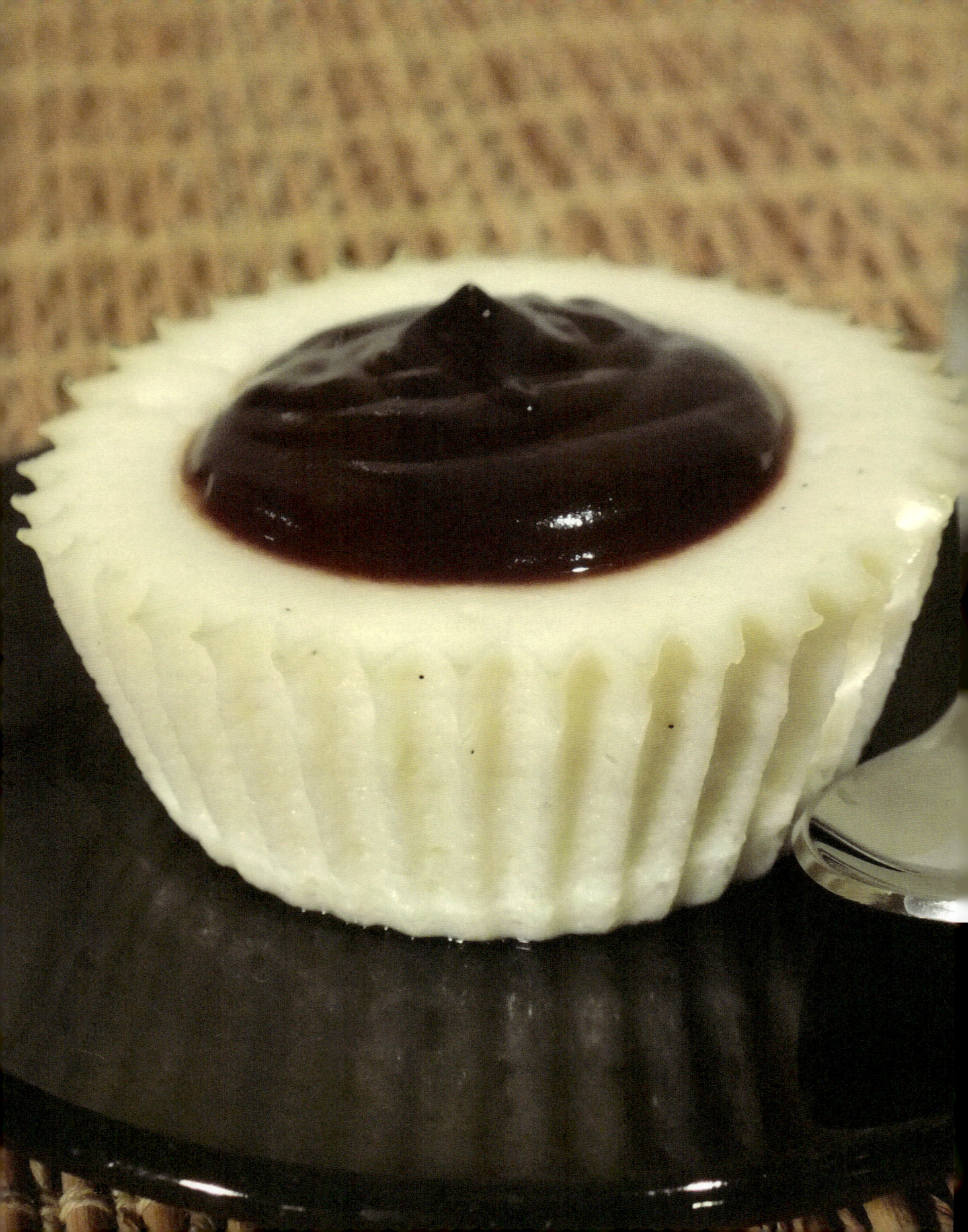

Chocolate-Cheese Cupcakes
Yield: 17 cupcakes | Per serving: 1cupcake - 160 calories

For the cupcakes:

1¾ cups (1 big container) ricotta cheese, part skim milk, 425 g, 600 calories

¾ cup Greek yogurt 2%, 180 g, 135 calories

¾ cup light sour cream, 180 g, 234 calories

4 extra-large eggs, 320 calories

1 cup granulated sugar, 200 g, 750 calories

½ teaspoon fine salt

1 tablespoon vanilla extract, 13 g, 37 calories

2 tablespoons all-purpose flour, 16 g, 54 calories

1 tablespoon cornstarch (corn flour), 8 g, 30 calories

For the chocolate topping:

½ cup of water plus 2 tablespoons

4 ounces semi-sweet chocolate, cut into ½-inch chunks (or ⅔ cup chocolate chips), 112 g, 560 calories

Preheat oven to 300°F (150°C).
Line a standard muffin tin with paper liners or baking cups, and spray with nonstick baking spray.
Put a pan (or any similar baking dish) with 1 cup of hot water on the bottom rack of the oven.

Cupcakes:
Combine the cheese, yogurt, sour cream, eggs, sugar, salt, and vanilla into a large bowl. Sift in the flour and cornstarch and combine.
Use an ice cream scoop to distribute the batter evenly among the baking cups, filling each 90 percent full. Bake for approximately one and a half hours. Cool in the pan for a few minutes before removing to a cooling rack. Refrigerate at least four hours.
Serve cold.
The cupcakes can be refrigerated up to three days in airtight containers.

Chocolate topping:
Add water to chocolate in a small saucepan over very low heat, and stir until chocolate is melted and mixture is completely smooth. Remove from heat and let cool approximately five minutes.
Just before serving, spoon about 1 teaspoon chocolate topping over each cupcake.

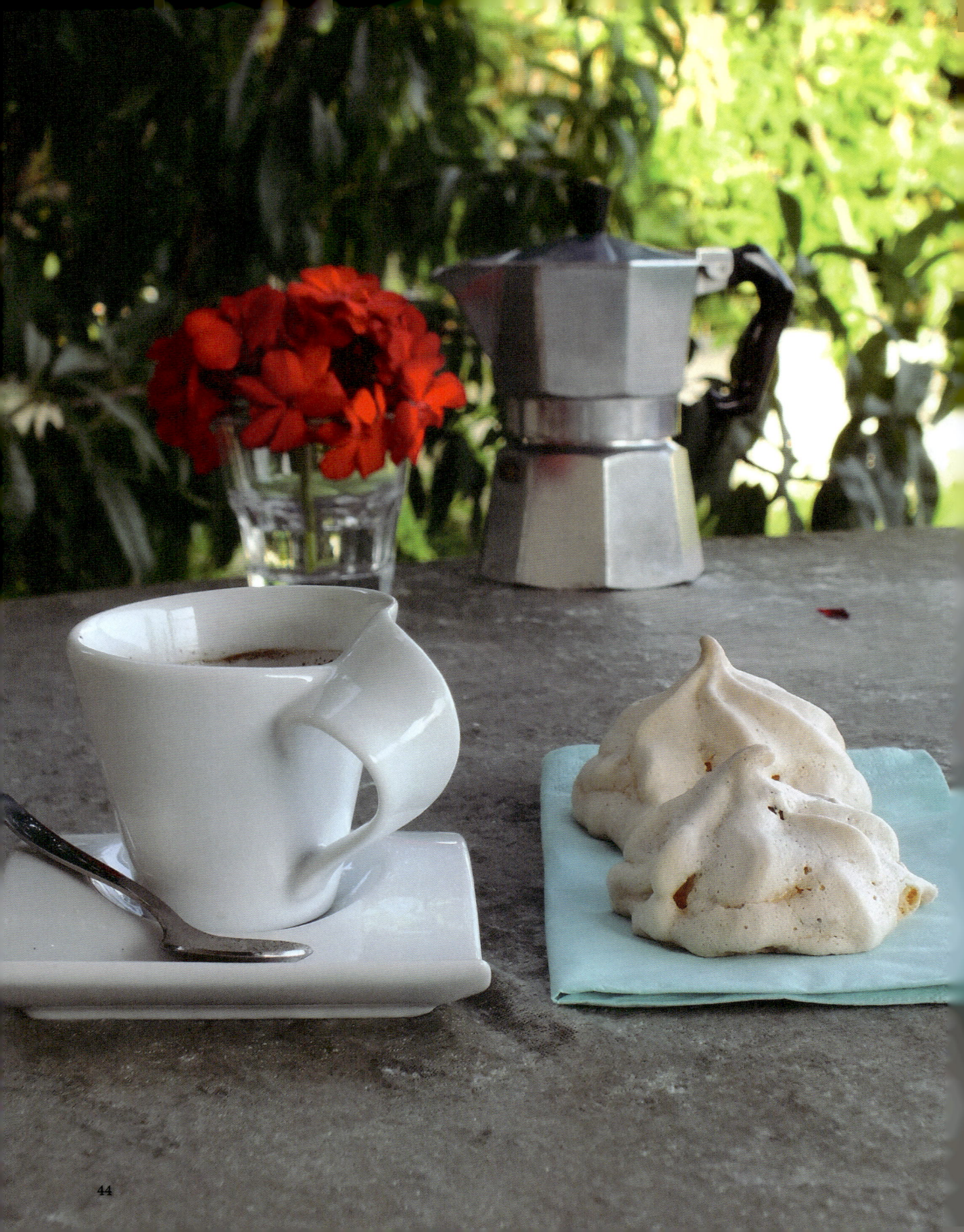

Chocolate-Almond Cookies

Yield: 30 cookies | Per serving: 2 cookies - 136 calories; 1 cookie - 68 calories

1 cup sliced or coarsely chopped almonds, 140 g, 813 calories

4 extra-large egg whites, 64 calories

½ teaspoon salt

1½ cup granulated sugar, 300 g, 1,125 calories

1½ teaspoons vanilla extract, 6 g, 18 calories

1 tablespoon cocoa powder, 5 g, 10 calories

Preheat oven to 300°F (150°C).
Line baking sheets with parchment paper, and spray with nonstick baking spray.
Place the almonds on a baking sheet, and bake for about five minutes or until fragrant. Remove from oven and let cool.

Combine egg whites and salt together in the bowl of an electric mixer—the bowl and beaters must be clean and free of grease—and beat on medium- high speed until soft peaks form (about four minutes). Add the sugar, a little at a time, and continue to beat until the meringue holds very stiff peaks. Beat in the vanilla extract and then sift in the cocoa powder. Lastly, fold in the almonds. Use an ice cream scoop or heaping tablespoonfuls to put batter about two inches apart onto prepared baking sheets.

Bake cookies for thirty minutes. Remove from oven and turn the oven to 250 F (120 C). When the oven comes to temperature, place the cookies back in the oven and bake for another thirty minutes. Remove from the oven and let cool to room temperature.
Cookies can be stored up to two days at room temperature in airtight containers.

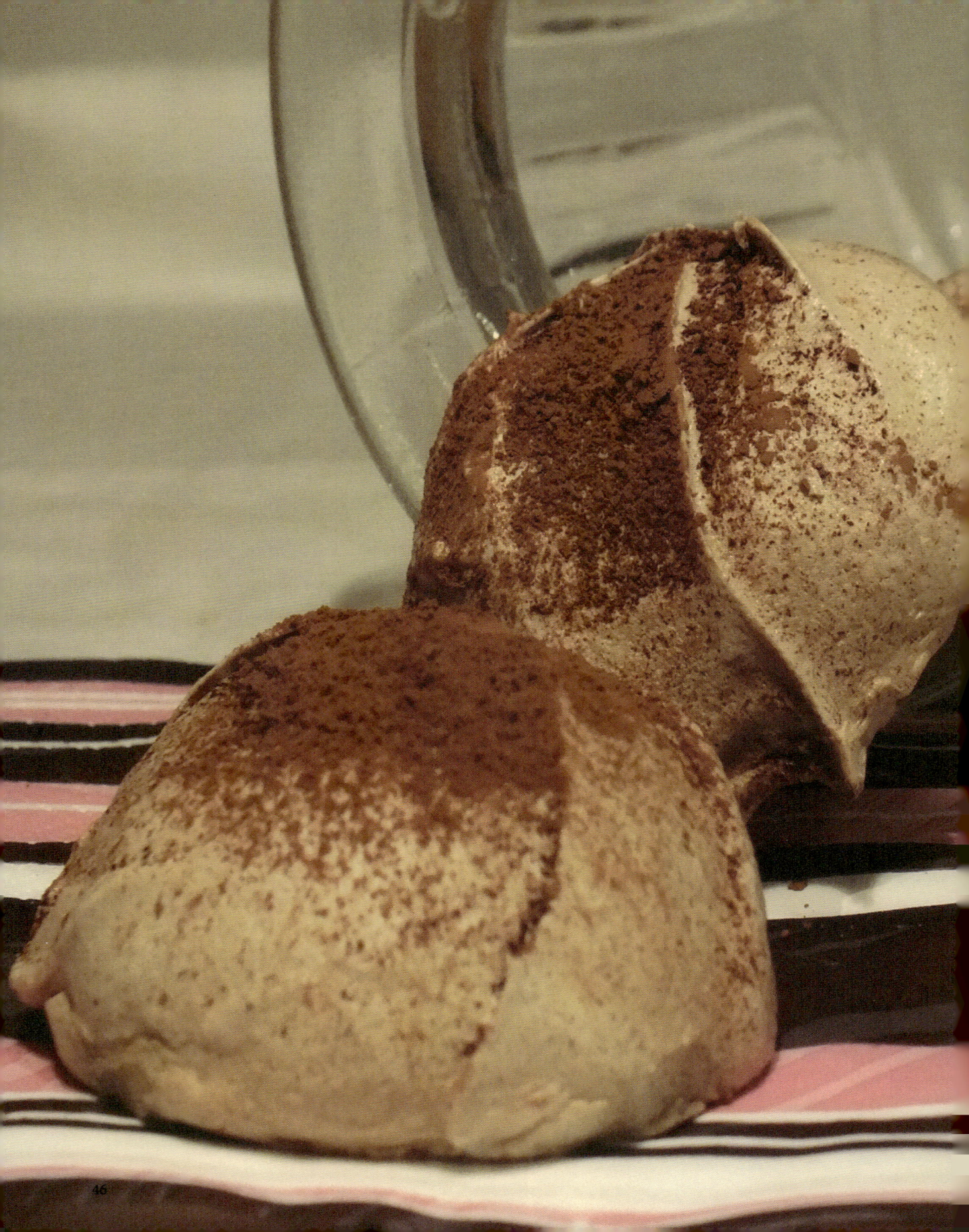

Cinnamon-Cocoa Meringue Cookies

Yield: 12 cookies | Per serving: 2 cookies - 108 calories; 1 cookie - 54 calories

2 extra-large egg whites, 32 calories

¼ teaspoon fine salt

1 teaspoon light corn syrup, 7 g, 21 calories

½ teaspoon white vinegar

¾ cup granulated sugar, 150 g, 562 calories

1 tablespoon cornstarch (corn flour), 8 g, 30 calories

1 teaspoon cocoa powder, 3 calories

¼ teaspoon cinnamon

Preheat oven to 230°F (110°C).
Line a baking sheet with parchment paper.

Combine egg whites, salt, light corn syrup, and white vinegar together in the bowl of an electric mixer—the bowl and beaters must be clean and free of grease—and beat on high speed until soft peaks form (about four minutes). Add the sugar, a little at a time, and continue to beat until the egg whites holds very stiff peaks.
Sift in the cornstarch, cocoa powder and the cinnamon and fold with a rubber spatula.
Use an ice cream scoop or heaping tablespoonfuls to put batter about two inches apart onto prepared baking sheets.

Bake for about two hours, rotating the baking sheet from front to back to ensure even baking. The meringues are done when they are fairly crisp. Turn off the heat and cool the meringues in the oven for an hour, propping the door open with a wooden spoon.
The meringues can be covered and stored up to two days at room temperature in airtight containers.

Berries

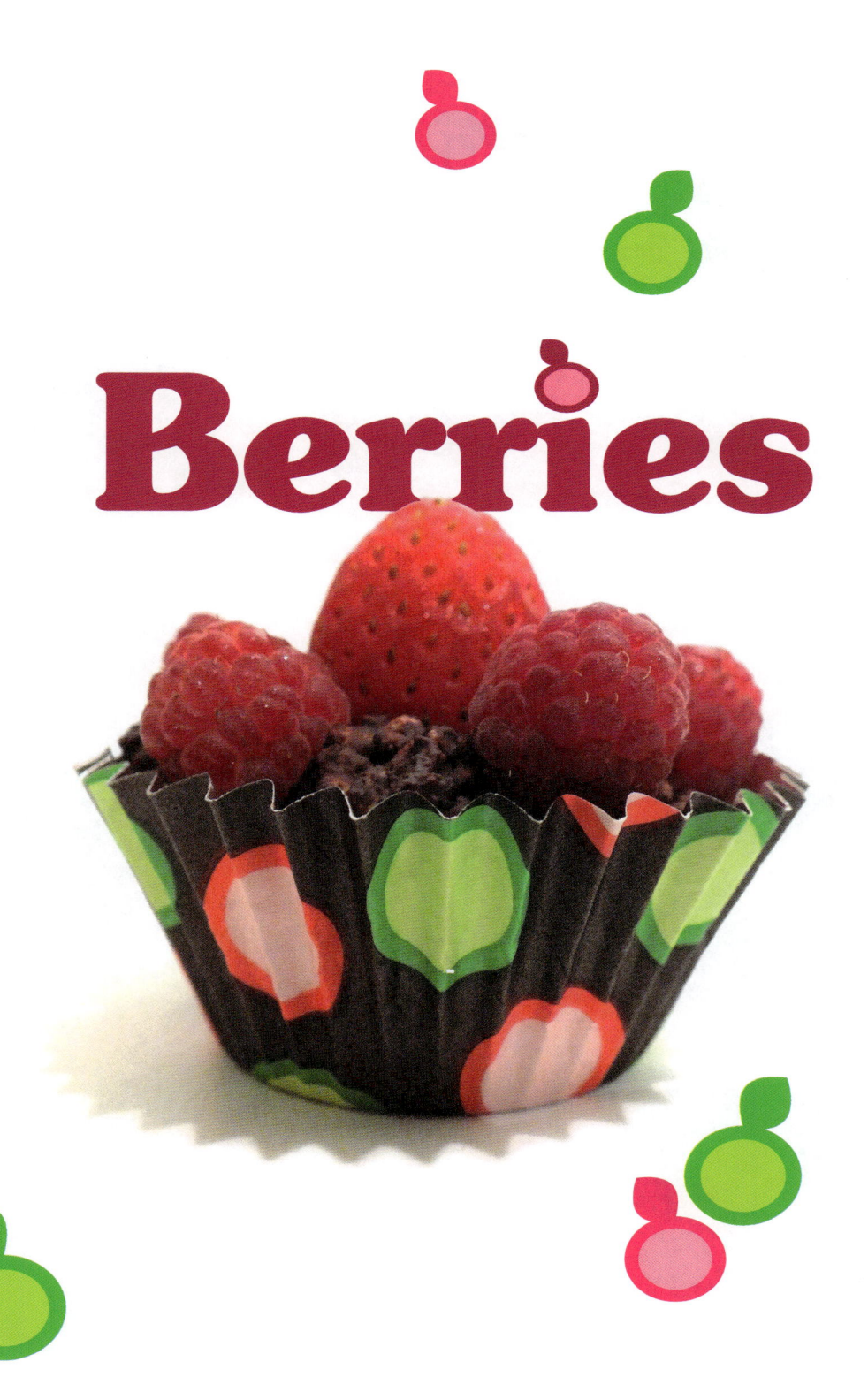

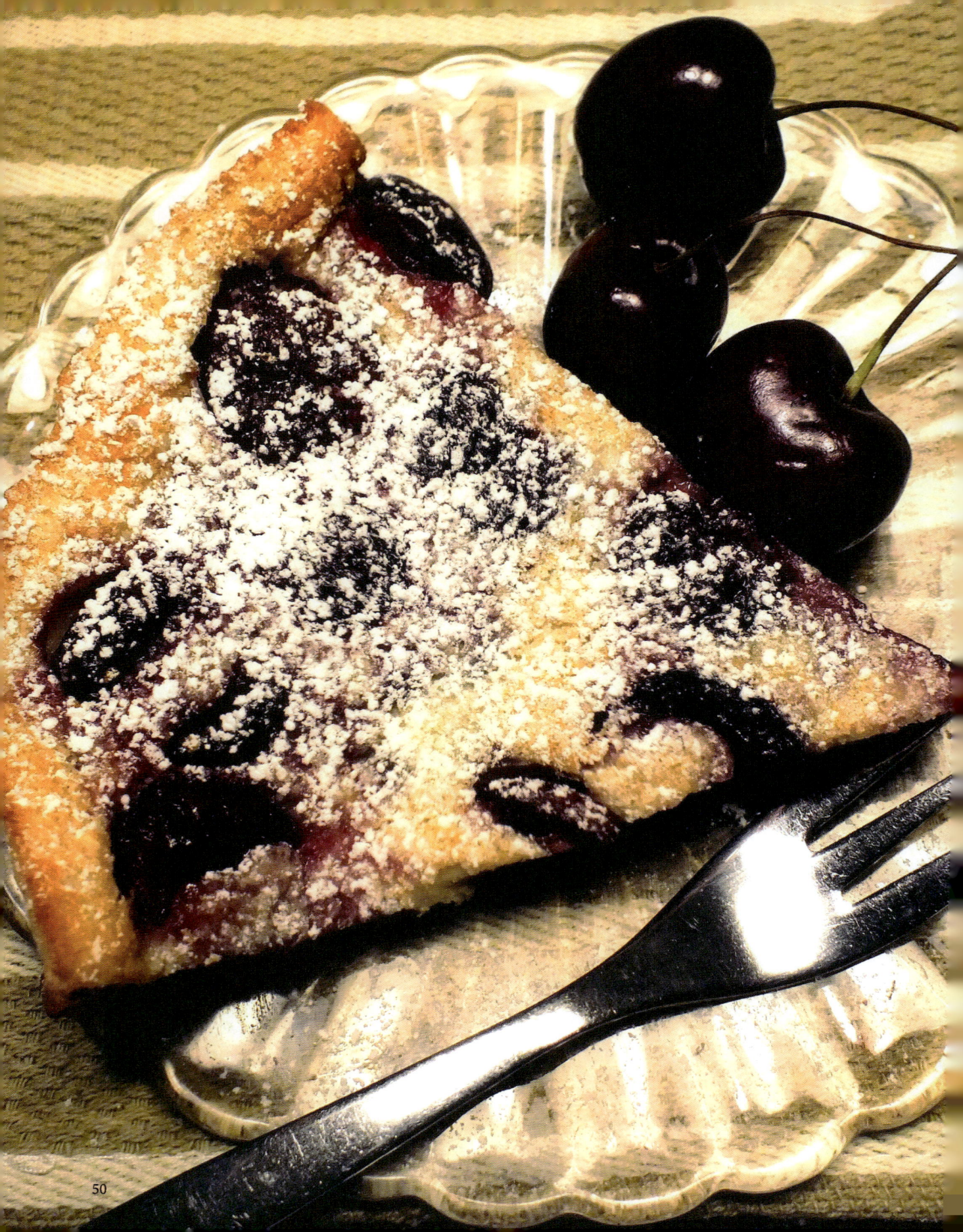

Cherry Clafouti
Yield: 7 | Per serving: 1/7 – 158 calories

1 tablespoon unsalted butter, 14 g, 100 calories

3 cups fresh sweet cherries pitted and cut in half, 1 pound, 454 g, 291 calories

4 tablespoons granulated sugar, 48 g, 180 calories

2 extra-large eggs, 160 calories

½ cup milk (1% fat), 120 ml, 54 calories

¼ cup water

½ teaspoon vanilla extract, 2 g, 6 calories

¼ teaspoon salt

½ cup all-purpose flour, 65 g, 217 calories

3 tablespoons powdered (confectioners') sugar, 24 g, 96 calories

Preheat oven to 350°F (175°C).
Place the rack in the center of the oven.

In a large nine- to ten-inch (twenty-three to twenty-five centimeters) nonstick ovenproof skillet, melt the butter over low heat, making sure the melted butter coats the bottom and sides of the pan. Add the pitted cherries and cook until the cherries have softened a bit and are coated with butter (about three minutes). Sprinkle the cherries with 4 tablespoons sugar, and cook until the sugar has dissolved and turned into a syrup (about two minutes). With an electric mixer, with the whisk attachment, beat the whole eggs on high speed until they are thick and fluffy (about two minutes).

In another bowl, combine the milk, water, vanilla, and salt. Sift in the flour and whisk until there are no lumps. Gently fold the flour mixture into the eggs until incorporated.

Pour the batter over the cherries and bake for about twenty-five to thirty minutes or until the clafouti is puffed and golden brown around the edges. Do not open the oven door until the end of the baking time, or it may collapse. To finish, dust with powdered (confectioners') sugar just before serving.
Serve immediately.

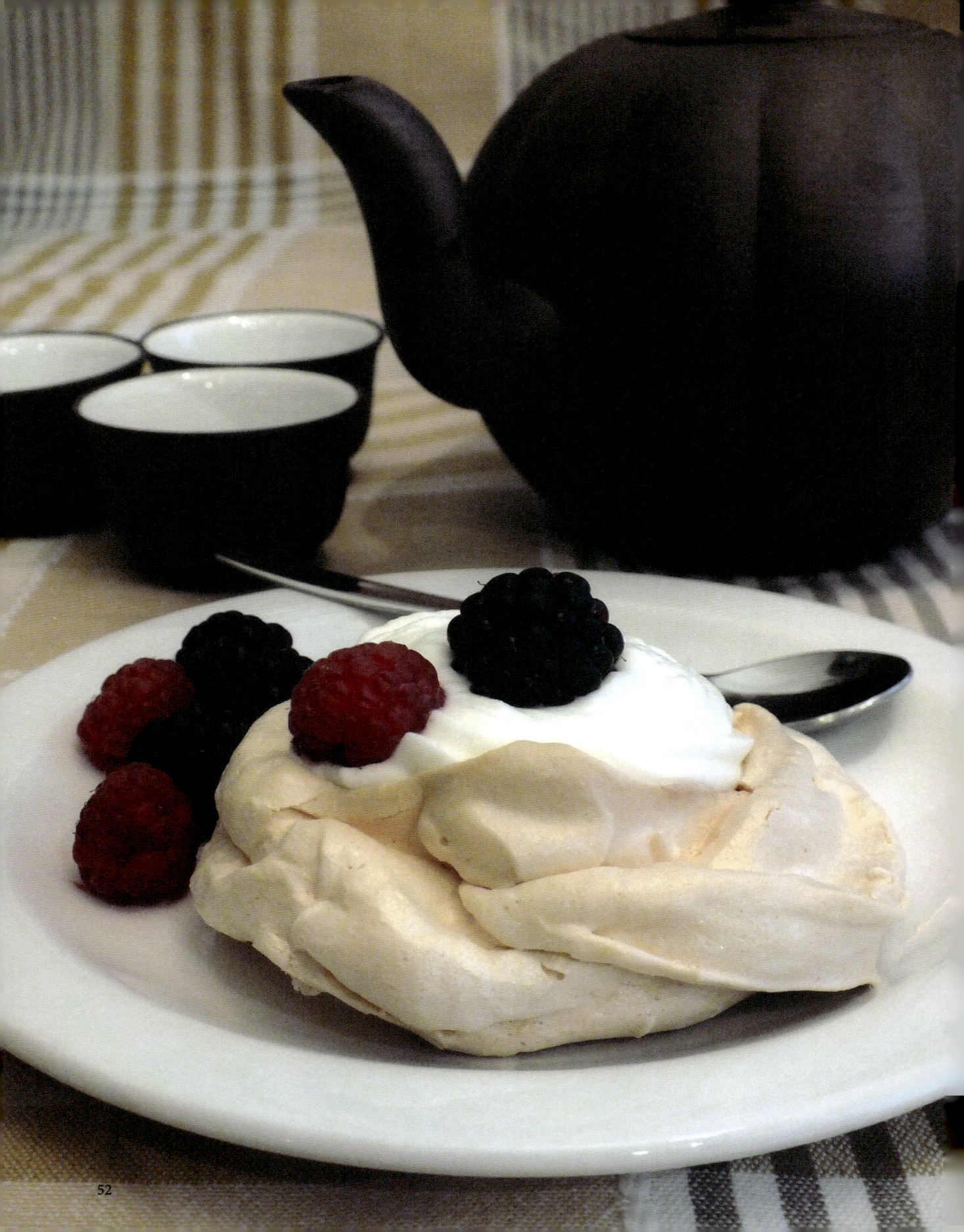

Berry Pavlova

Yield: 6 Pavlovas | Per serving: 1 Pavlova – 160 calories

For the Pavlovas:

2 extra-large egg whites, 32 calories

Pinch fine salt

¼ teaspoon white vinegar

½ cup granulated sugar, 100 g, 375 calories

¼ teaspoon vanilla extract, 3 calories

1½ teaspoons cornstarch (corn flour), 4 g, 15 calories

For the cream:

½ cup heavy cream (double cream), 120 ml, 400 calories

1½ tablespoons granulated sugar, 18 g, 67 calories

1 teaspoon instant vanilla pudding, 3 g, 12 calories

¾ cup fresh berries, 105 g, 60 calories

Preheat oven to 250°F (130°C).

Combine egg whites, salt, and white vinegar together in the bowl of an electric mixer and beat on high speed until soft peaks form. Add the sugar, a little at a time, and continue to beat until the egg whites holds very stiff peaks. Add the vanilla extract and beat until stiff peaks form. Sift in the cornstarch and fold with a rubber spatula.

Line a baking sheet with parchment paper and spoon the meringue in six big spoonfuls, using a spoon to spread them in a circle, and then make an indent in each. Bake for about two hours. Turn off the heat and cool the meringues in the oven for an hour, propping the door open with a wooden spoon.

Meanwhile, place the heavy cream, the remaining 1½ tablespoons of sugar, and the instant pudding in the bowl of your electric mixer. With the whisk attachment, whip the cream until soft peaks form. Do not overbeat.

Just before serving:

Evenly distribute the cream on the meringues, filling in the indentations. Top with berries, and serve.

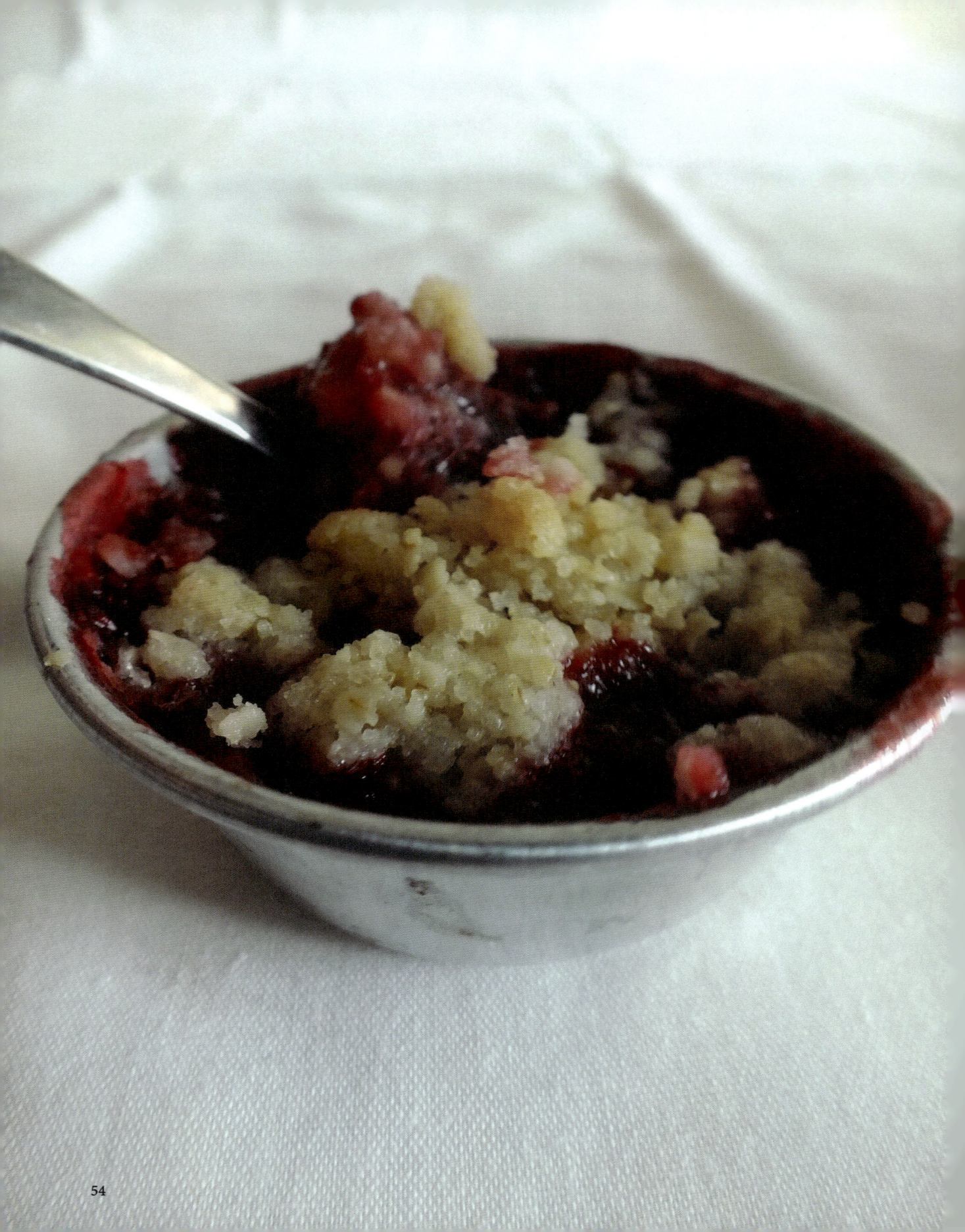

Berry-Oat Crumble

Yield: 6 crumbles | Per serving: 1 crumble – 157 calories

For the topping:

3 tablespoons all-purpose flour, 24 g, 81 calories

6 tablespoons granulated sugar, 72 g, 270 calories

3 tablespoons quick cooking white oats, 18 g, 64 calories

½ teaspoon baking powder

3 tablespoons unsalted butter, 42 g, 300 calories

For the crumble:

2 tablespoons granulated sugar, 24 g, 90 calories

1½ teaspoons cornstarch (corn flour), 4 g, 15 calories

1½ cups fresh berries (blueberries, strawberries, raspberries), 210 g, 120 calories

Special equipment: Six 2.5- to 3-ounce (80 ml) ramekins

Combine the flour, 6 tablespoons sugar, oats, and baking powder in a small bowl. Cut the butter into small pieces and blend into the flour mixture with a pastry blender or two knives or a spoon. The mixture should look like crumbs. Refrigerate at least thirty minutes before using.

Preheat the oven to 350°F (175°C).
In a medium bowl, combine the 2 tablespoons sugar and the cornstarch. Add the berries and combine.
Pour evenly into the ramekins and then spread the topping over the fruit. Bake for about forty minutes or until the topping is browned and the fruit juices are bubbling.

Serve immediately.
Refrigerate leftovers and reheat before serving.

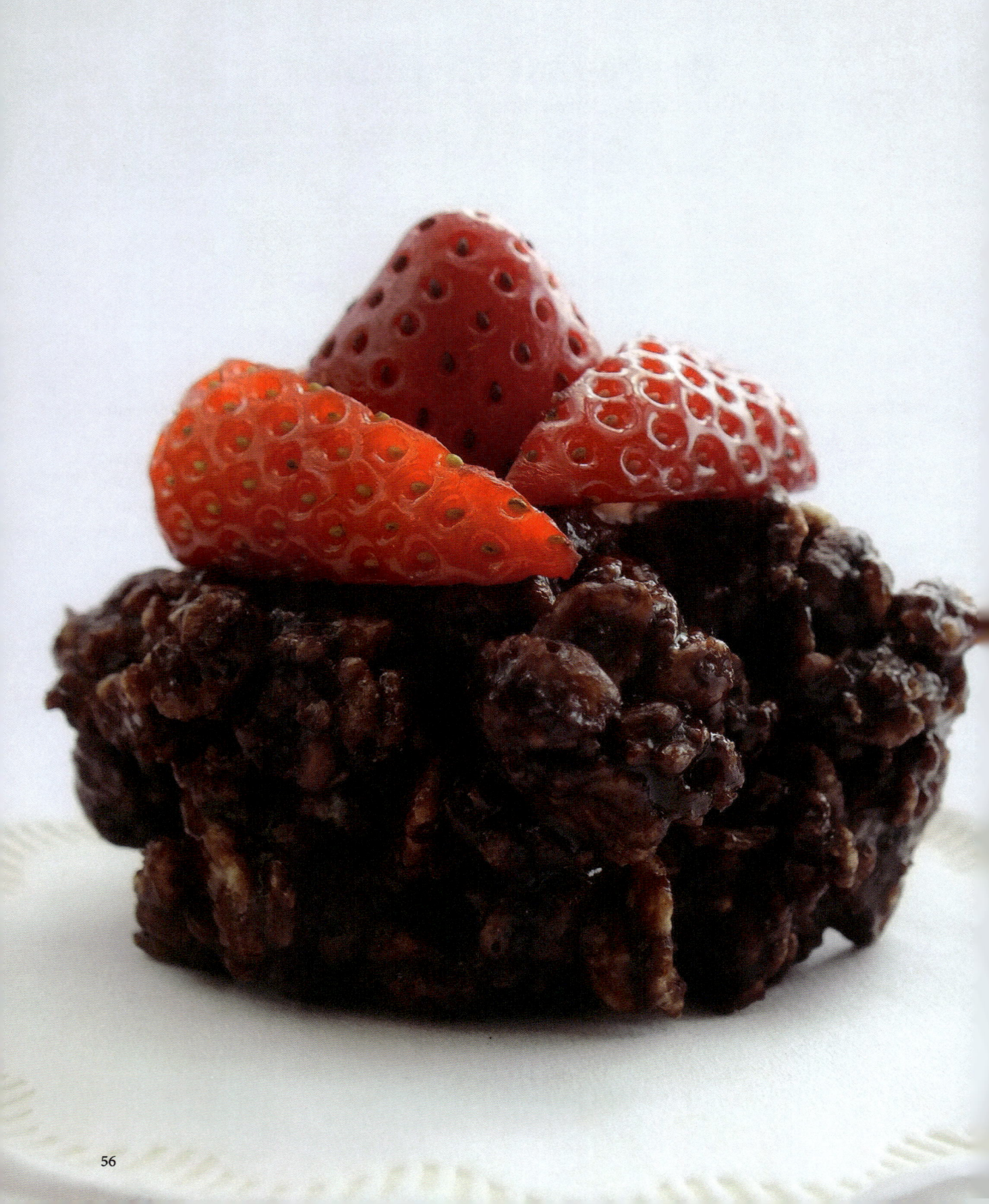

Chocolate-Berry Rice Krispies Treats

Yield: 12 treats | Per serving: 1 treat – 148 calories

3¾ cups Rice Krispies, 100 g,
390 calories

¼ cup plus 1 tablespoon of water

9 ounces semi-sweet chocolate,
cut into ½-inch chunks (or 1½
cups chocolate chips), 252 g,
1,260 calories

12 strawberries (about 120 g),
38 calories

48 raspberries (about 180 g),
94 calories

Line standard muffin tin with baking cups and spray with nonstick spray.

Put the Rice Krispies in a large mixing bowl.
Add water to chocolate in a small saucepan over very low heat, and stir until chocolate is melted and mixture is completely smooth. Remove from heat and let cool approximately five minutes. Pour into Rice Krispies and mix together quickly. Using two spoons, distribute into baking cups.

Press down gently on each and top off with strawberries and raspberries. Cover the tin loosely with a plastic bag and freeze at least one hour.
Box them up and keep in the refrigerator for up to two days.

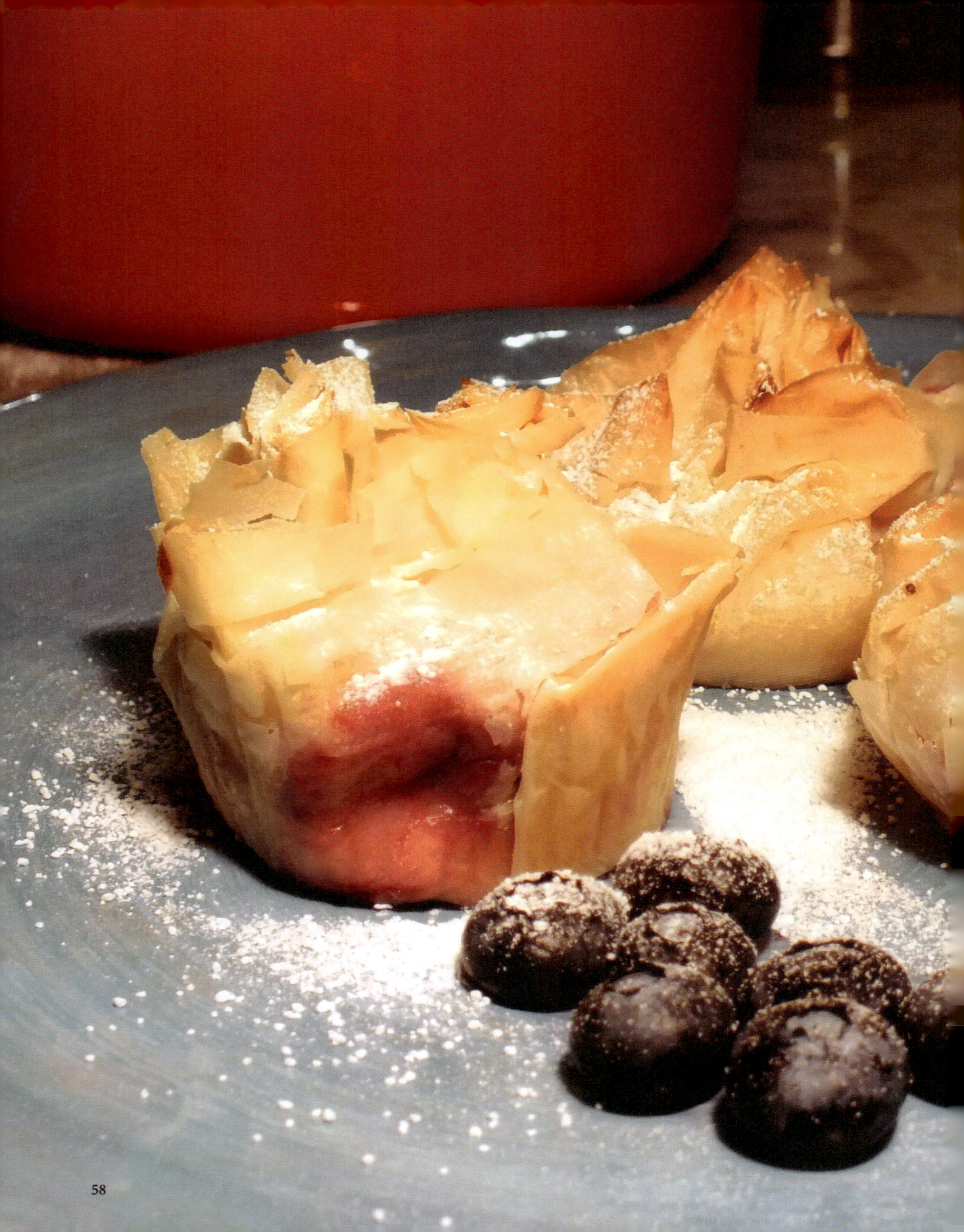

Berry and Cheese Strudel

Yield: 16 strudels | Per serving: 1 strudel – 142 calories

1 cup Greek yogurt 2%, 240 g, 180 calories

¾ cup ricotta cheese, part-skim milk, 185 g, 257 calories

1 cup granulated sugar, 200 g, 750 calories

2 extra-large eggs, 160 calories

¾ teaspoon finely grated lemon zest

1½ teaspoons vanilla extract, 6 g, 18 calories

½ teaspoon fine salt

4 tablespoons all-purpose flour, 32 g, 108 calories

2 cups fresh berries (blueberries or cherries pitted and sliced in half), 280 g, 160 calories

Butter-flavored nonstick baking spray, 75 calories

16 sheets of phyllo (fillo) pastry. Sheet size 9"x14" (22x35 cm) is preferable (I used Athens brand), though you can cut other sizes, 182 g, 512 calories

1½ tablespoons powdered (confectioners') sugar, 12 g, 48 calories

Combine the yogurt, cheese, sugar, eggs, lemon zest, vanilla, and salt in a large bowl. Sift in the flour and then fold in the blueberries/chopped cherries.
Preheat oven to 350°F (175°C).

Line a standard muffin tin with paper liners (or baking cups) and spray with nonstick baking spray.
Open the phyllo pastry sheets and layer one phyllo sheet, lightly coating with butter-flavored nonstick baking spray. Make sure to keep the unbuttered phyllo covered with a damp towel.
To prevent edges from cracking, spray edges first and then work into center. Fold the sheet in half and spray again. Fold it again; the sheet is now one-quarter of its original size.

Place into the muffin cup. Carefully push phyllo into cup, pressing firmly against bottom and sides (do not worry if the phyllo tears a little bit). Repeat fifteen times to make sixteen shells. Spoon cheese mixture into phyllo and gather points to close the phyllo. Spray again. Bake until golden brown, ten to twenty minutes.
Cool in the pan for a few minutes before removing to a cooling rack.
To finish, dust with powdered (confectioners') sugar just before serving.
Best served at room temperature.

Note:
There are two important things about phyllo: 1) Get everything ready before opening the packet of pastry; once the phyllo is open, it will dry quickly; 2) Cover phyllo completely with plastic wrap, then a damp towel.

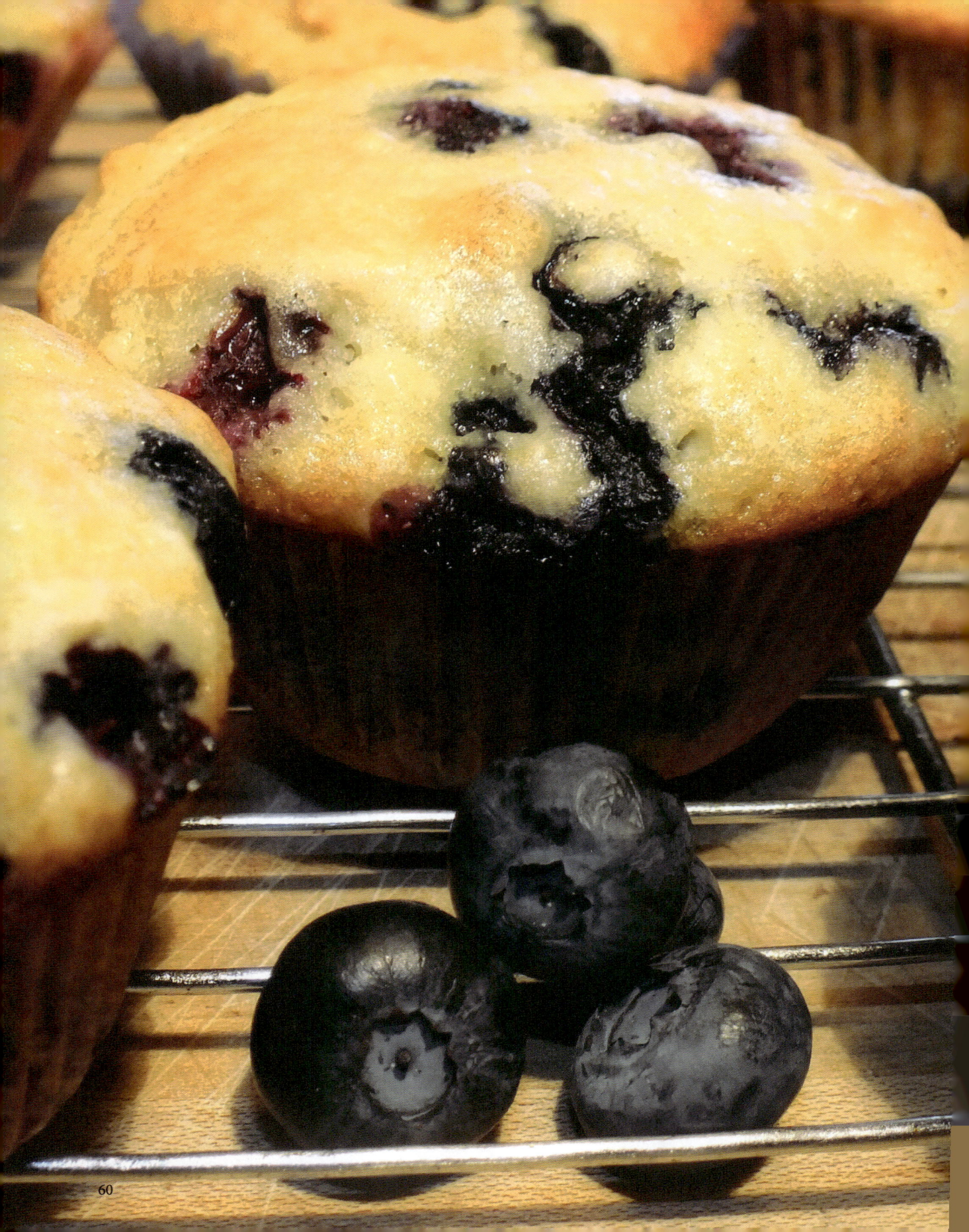

Blueberry Muffins with Orange Juice Syrup

Yield: 16 muffins | Per serving: 1 muffin – 156 calories

For the blueberry muffins:

2 cups all-purpose flour, 260 g, 866 calories

2 teaspoons baking powder

1 teaspoon baking soda

1 cup granulated sugar, 200 g, 750 calories

¼ cup unsweetened applesauce, 52 g, 21 calories

¾ cup Greek yogurt 2%, 180 g, 135 calories

1 teaspoon vanilla extract, 4 g, 12 calories

3 extra-large eggs, 240 calories

¼ teaspoon salt

2 tablespoons unsalted butter, melted and cooled, 28 g, 200 calories

2 cups fresh blueberries, 280 g, 160 calories

For the orange juice syrup:

½ cup orange juice, 120 ml, 54 calories

2 tablespoons powdered sugar, 16 g, 64 calories

Preheat oven to 350°F (175°C).

Line a standard muffin tin with paper liners (or baking cups) and spray with nonstick baking spray.

Put a pan (or any similar baking dish) with 1 cup of water on the bottom rack of the oven.

Sift flour, baking powder, and baking soda into a medium-sized bowl. Mix in the sugar.

Puree the applesauce in a blender or a food processor (the applesauce needs to be finely pureed and smooth) and then measure ¼ cup.

Combine the Greek yogurt, applesauce, and vanilla in a separate bowl.

With an electric mixer, with the whisk attachment, beat the whole eggs on low speed for a minute then add the salt. Increase the speed to high and gradually add the butter until the batter is thick and fluffy (about two minutes).

Gently fold the yogurt/applesauce mixture into the eggs until incorporated.

Make a well in the dry ingredients and pour in the liquid mixture then fold in the blueberries. Stir just to combine (do not over-mix or you will have tough muffins).

Use an ice cream scoop to distribute the batter evenly among the baking cups, filling each 90 percent full. Bake for approximately twenty to twenty-five minutes or until a toothpick tests clean or with a few crumbs. Cool in the pan for a few minutes before removing to a cooling rack.

Meanwhile, stirring constantly, heat the orange juice and the powdered sugar in a saucepan to dissolve the sugar, but do not boil. Remove from heat and let cool for about five minutes before pouring equally onto the muffins.

Muffins can be stored up to two days in the refrigerator.

Cranberry Raisin Biscotti

Yield: 40 biscotti | Per serving: 2 biscotti – 134 calories; 1 biscotto – 67 calories

2½ cups all-purpose flour, 325 g, 1,083 calories

2 teaspoons baking powder

1 teaspoon ground cinnamon, 2 g, 6 calories

1¼ cups granulated sugar, 250 g, 938 calories

¼ teaspoon salt

3 extra-large eggs, 240 calories

1 teaspoon vanilla extract, 4 g, 12 calories

½ cup raisins, 70 g, 198 calories

½ cup dried cranberries, sweetened, 70 g, 215 calories

Preheat oven to 350°F (175°C).
Line a baking sheet with parchment paper.
In the bowl of an electric mixer, combine the flour, baking powder, cinnamon, sugar, and salt. In another small bowl, whisk the eggs and the vanilla. Gradually add the egg mixture to the flour and beat until a dough forms, adding raisins and cranberries about halfway through. If the dough does not form add one to three tablespoons of water.

With floured hands (the dough is quite sticky), divide the dough into two pieces. On a lightly floured surface, roll each half of the dough into a log about sixteen inches (forty centimeters) long and two inches (five centimeters) wide. Transfer the logs to the prepared baking sheet, spacing about four inches (ten centimeters) apart. Logs will spread during baking. Bake until firm to the touch, about twenty-five to thirty minutes. Let cool for about twenty minutes.

Reduce oven temperature to 300°F (150°C).
Cut the logs into slices about ½-inch (1¼ cm) thick using a serrated knife; cut each log into twenty pieces. Arrange the slices, cut side down, on the baking sheet and bake ten minutes. Then turn slices over and bake another ten minutes or until golden brown. Remove from oven and let cool on a wire rack.
Cookies can be stored in an airtight container for a month.

Blueberry Streusel Muffins

Yield: 15 muffins | Per serving: 1 muffin – 151 calories

For the streusel topping:

2 tablespoons all-purpose flour, 18 g, 54 calories

2 tablespoons granulated sugar, 24 g, 90 calories

⅛ teaspoon baking powder

1 tablespoon unsalted butter, 14 g, 100 calories

For the muffins:

1¼ cups all-purpose flour, 166 g, 542 calories

1¼ teaspoons baking powder

¾ cup granulated sugar, 150 g, 562 calories

3 extra-large eggs, 240 calories

¾ cup Greek yogurt 2%, 180 g, 135 calories

2 tablespoons vegetable oil, 28 g, 248 calories

2 tablespoons honey, 42 g, 128 calories

1 teaspoon vanilla extract, 4 g, 12 calories

¼ teaspoon fine salt

2 cups fresh blueberries, 280 g, 160 calories

For the streusel topping, combine the flour, sugar, and baking powder in a small bowl. Cut the butter into small pieces and blend into the flour mixture with a pastry blender or a spoon to form crumbs. Refrigerate at least thirty minutes before using.

Preheat oven to 350°F (175°C).

Line a standard muffin tin with paper liners (or baking cups) and spray with nonstick baking spray.

Sift the flour and the baking powder into a medium-sized bowl. Mix in the sugar.

In another large bowl, whisk together eggs, yogurt, oil, honey, vanilla, and salt.

Make a well in the flour mixture, pour in the liquid mixture, and fold in the blueberries. Stir just to combine (do not over-mix or you will have tough muffins).

Divide batter evenly among lined cups, filling each ¾ full, then sprinkle the streusel topping evenly.

Bake for approximately twenty to twenty-five minutes. Cool in the pan for a few minutes before removing to a cooling rack.

Muffins can be stored up to two days at room temperature in airtight containers.

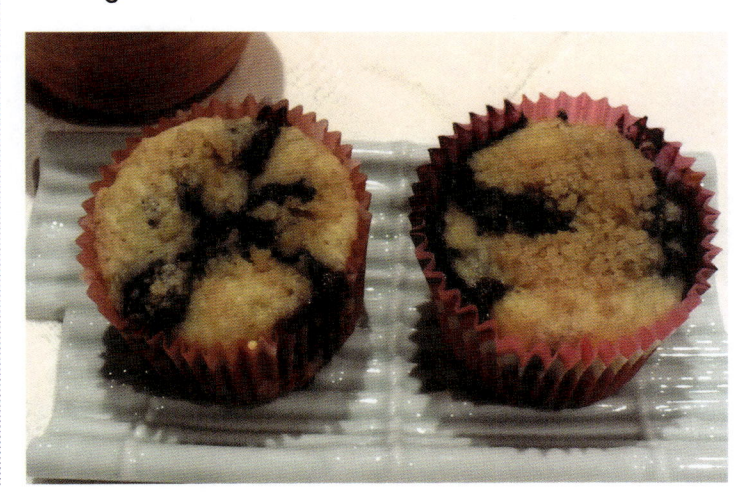

Chocolate-Berry Meringue Cupcakes
Yield: 17 cupcakes | Per serving: 1 cupcake – 146 calories

For the cupcakes:

5 tablespoons of water

4 ounces semi-sweet chocolate, cut into ½ inch chunks (or ⅔ cup chocolate chips), 112 g, 560 calories

¾ cup all-purpose flour, 98 g, 325 calories

1 tablespoon cocoa powder, 5 g, 10 calories

¾ teaspoon baking powder

¾ teaspoon baking soda

½ cup granulated sugar, 100 g, 375 calories

½ cup unsweetened applesauce, 105 g, 43 calories

¾ cup Greek yogurt 2%, 180 g, 135 calories

1 teaspoon vanilla extract, 4 g, 12 calories

½ cup milk (1% fat), 120 ml, 54 calories

1 extra-large egg, 80 calories

3 extra-large egg yolks, 192 calories

¼ teaspoon fine salt

1 cup fresh berries (blueberries, raspberries, or sweet cherries, pitted), 140 g, 80 calories

For the meringue:

2 egg whites at room temperature, 32 calories

¼ teaspoon fine salt

¾ cup granulated sugar, 150 g, 562 calories

½ teaspoon vanilla extract, 2 g, 6 calories

1 tablespoon cocoa powder, 5 g, 10 calories

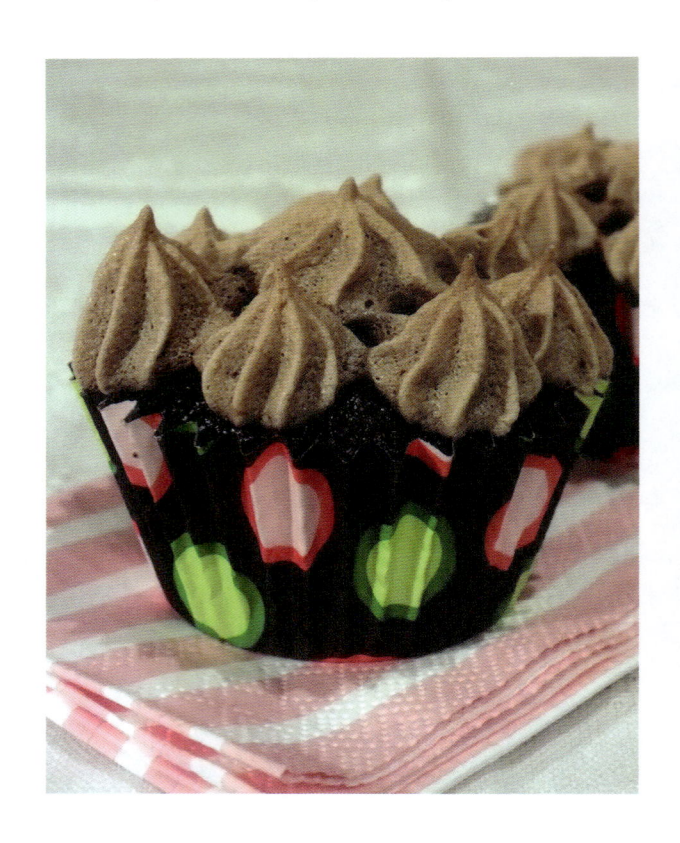

Preheat oven to 340°F (170°C).

Line a standard muffin tin with paper liners (or baking cups) and spray with nonstick baking spray.

Put a pan (or any similar baking dish) with 1 cup of water on the bottom rack of the oven.

Add water to chocolate in a small saucepan over very low heat, and stir until chocolate is melted and mixture is completely smooth. Remove from heat and let cool approximately five minutes.

Sift the flour, cocoa, baking powder, and baking soda together in a large mixing bowl. Mix in the sugar.

Puree the applesauce in a blender or a food processor (the applesauce needs to be finely pureed and smooth) and then measure ½ cup.

In a medium bowl, whisk together the yogurt, vanilla, applesauce, milk, and chocolate mixture. Stir until the mixture is combined and smooth.

With an electric mixer, with the whisk attachment, beat the whole egg, 3 egg yolks, and the salt on high speed until the batter is thick and fluffy (about two minutes).

Gently fold the yogurt/chocolate mixture into the eggs until incorporated.

Make a well in the flour mixture, and pour in the liquid mixture. Stir just to combine and fold in the berries (do not over-mix or you will have tough cupcakes).

Use an ice cream scoop to distribute the batter evenly among the baking cups, filling each 90 percent full. Bake for approximately twenty-five minutes, until firm but not fully baked.

Make the meringue when the cupcakes are in the oven.

With an electric mixer—the bowl and beaters must be clean and free of grease—beat the egg whites on medium-high speed until foamy. Add the salt and continue to beat until they hold soft peaks. Add the sugar, a little at a time, and continue to beat until the meringue holds very stiff peaks. Beat in the vanilla extract. Sift cocoa over the egg whites and gently fold in until just blended. Transfer meringue to pastry bag fitted with a small open-star tip.

Remove the cupcakes from the oven and pipe five to seven starbursts around the perimeter of the warm cupcakes, then pipe another starburst in the center. Return to the oven and bake about five minutes. Do not over-bake or you will have dry cupcakes.

Cool in the pan for a few minutes before removing to a cooling rack.

Cupcakes can be refrigerated up to two days in airtight containers.

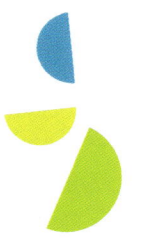

Apples
Bananas
Plums

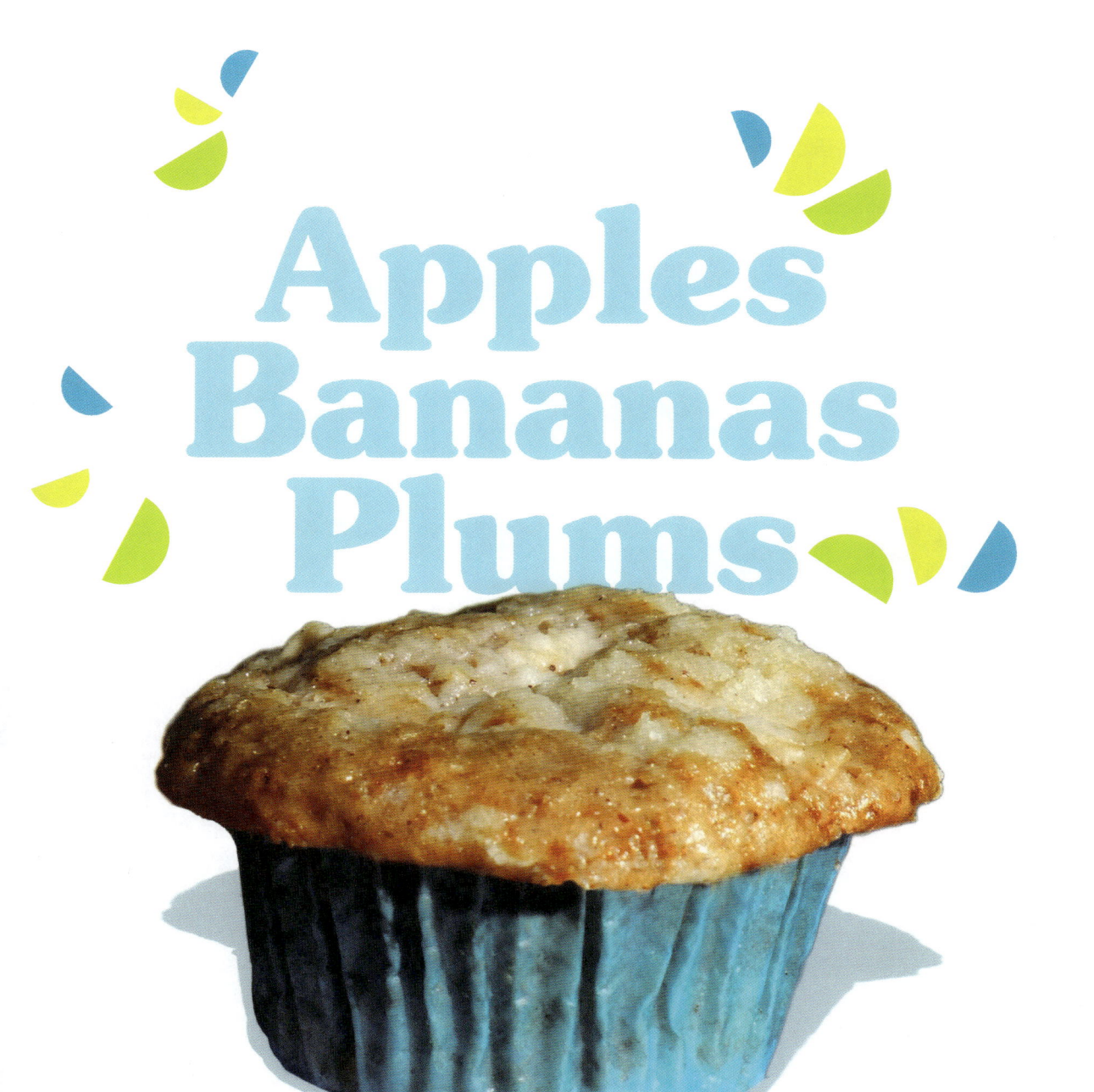

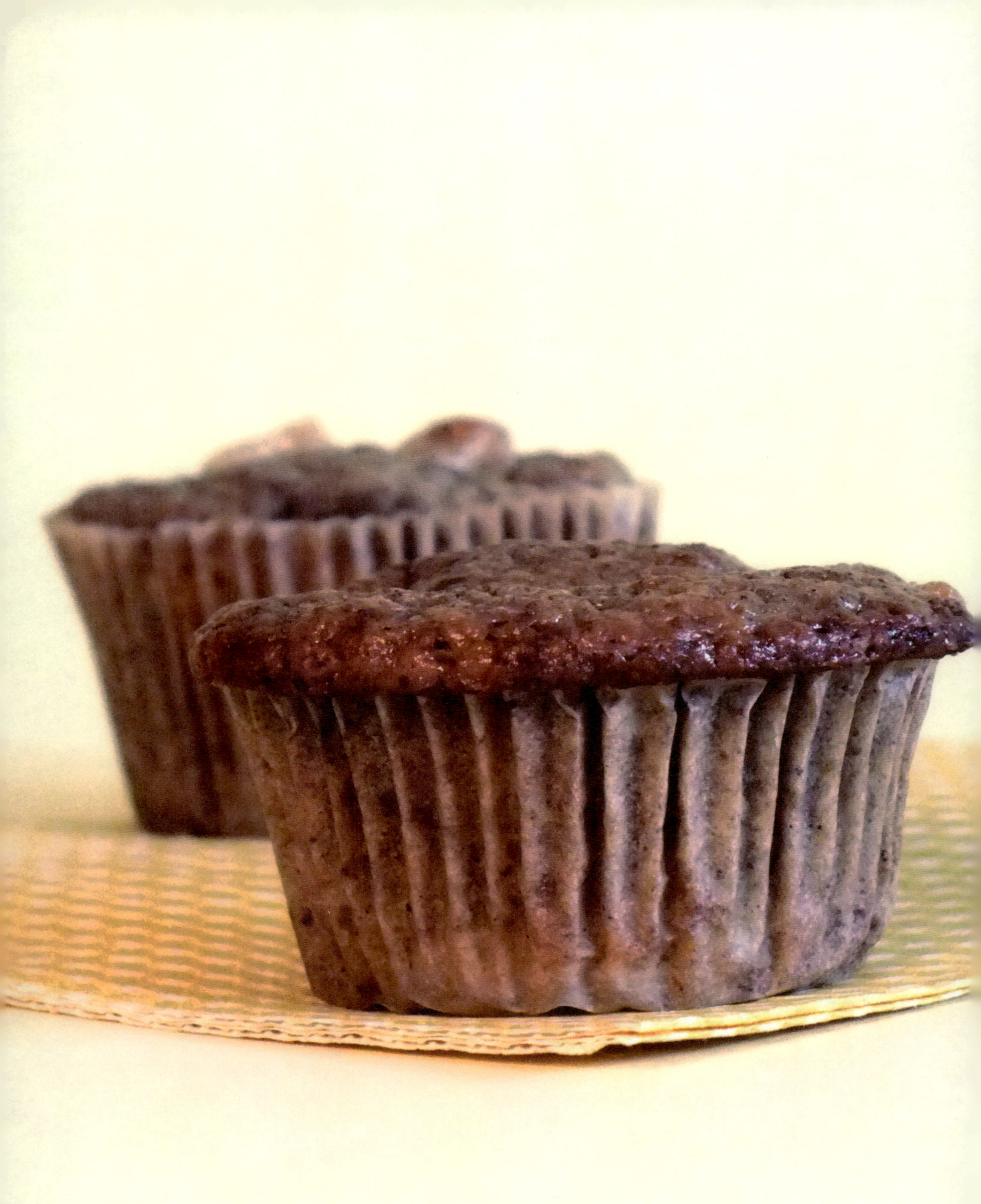

Apple Muffins
Yield: 18 muffins | Per serving: 1 muffin – 124 calories

For the muffins:

1½ cups all-purpose flour, 195 g, 650 calories

1½ teaspoons baking powder

½ teaspoon baking soda

1 cup granulated sugar, 200 g, 750 calories

2 teaspoons ground cinnamon, 4 g, 12 calories

1 cup unsweetened applesauce, 210 g, 86 calories

3 extra-large eggs, 240 calories

¾ cup Greek yogurt 2%, 180 g, 135 calories

½ teaspoon finely grated lemon zest

½ teaspoon fine salt

1 teaspoon vanilla extract, 4 g, 12 calories

4 cups apples, peeled, cored and cut into ¼-inch (½ cm) slices, about 480 g, 264 calories

For the topping:

2 tablespoons sugar, 24 g, 90 calories

¼ teaspoon cinnamon

Preheat oven to 350°F (175°C).

Line standard muffin tin with baking cups and spray with nonstick spray.

Sift the flour, baking powder, and baking soda together in a large mixing bowl. Mix in the sugar and the cinnamon. Puree the applesauce in a blender or a food processor (the applesauce needs to be finely pureed and smooth) and then measure 1 cup.

In a medium bowl, whisk together the eggs, Greek yogurt, lemon zest, applesauce, salt, and vanilla.

Mix together the topping ingredients into a small bowl. Make a well in the flour mixture, and pour in the liquid mixture. Fold in the apples. Stir just to combine (do not over-mix or you will have tough muffins).

Use an ice cream scoop to distribute the batter evenly among the baking cups, filling each 90 percent full, and then sprinkle evenly the sugar and the cinnamon topping.

Bake for approximately twenty-five to thirty minutes or until a toothpick tests clean or with a few crumbs (do not over-bake or you will have dry muffins). Cool in the pan for a few minutes before removing to a cooling rack. Muffins can be stored up to three days in the refrigerator. Reheat in microwave.

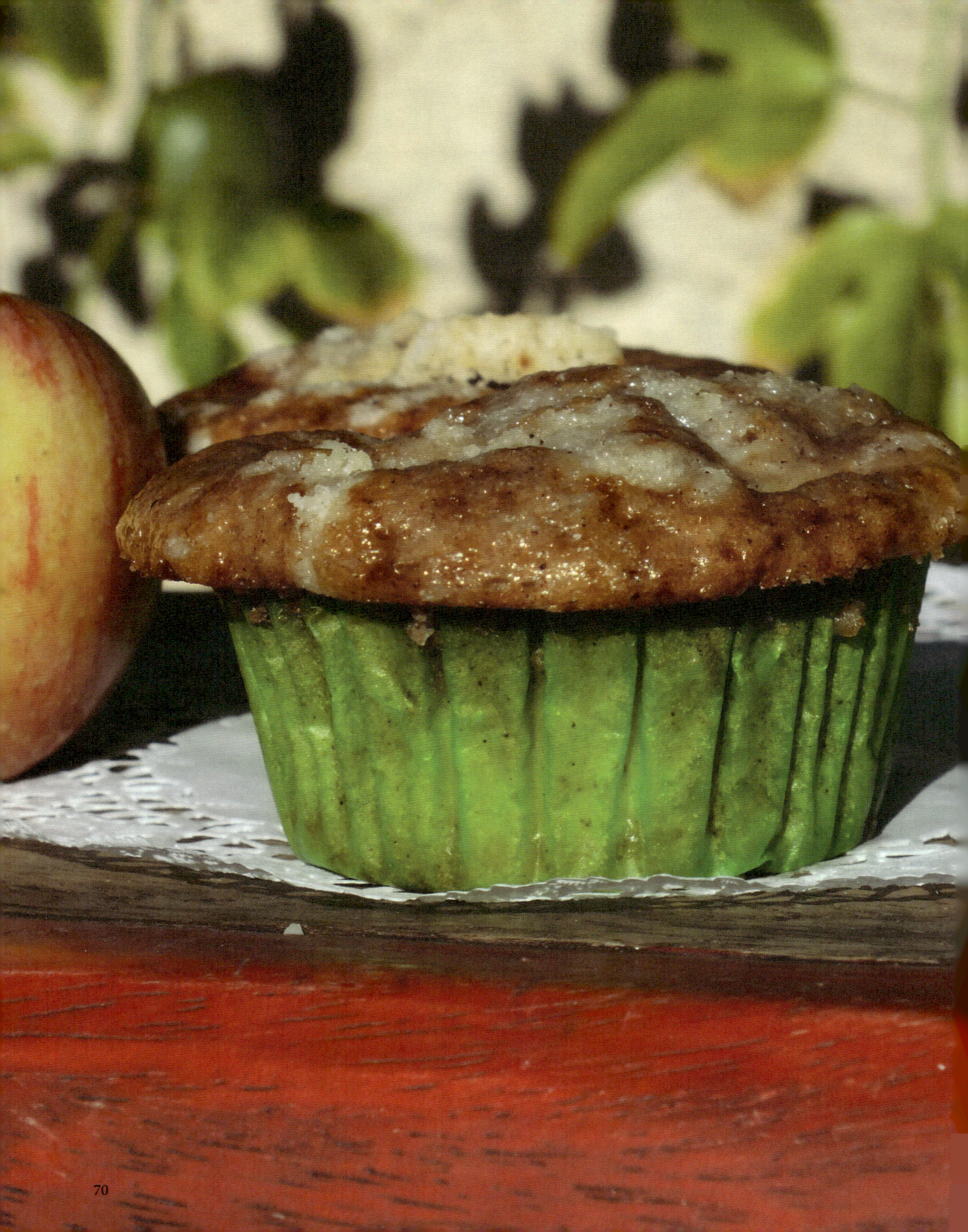

Streusel Apple Muffins
Yield: 16 muffins | Per serving: 1 muffin – 149 calories

For the streusel topping:

2 tablespoons all-purpose flour, 16 g, 54 calories

2 tablespoons granulated sugar, 24 g, 90 calories

⅛ teaspoon baking powder

⅛ teaspoon cinnamon

1 tablespoon unsalted butter, 14 g, 100 calories

For the muffins:

1 cup unsweetened applesauce, 210 g, 86 calories

1½ cups all-purpose flour, 195 g, 650 calories

1½ teaspoons baking powder

½ teaspoon baking soda

1 cup granulated sugar, 200 g, 750 calories

1 teaspoon ground cinnamon, 2 g, 6 calories

3 extra-large eggs, 240 calories

¾ cup Greek yogurt 2%, 180 g, 135 calories

½ teaspoon finely grated lemon zest

½ teaspoon fine salt

1 teaspoon vanilla extract, 4 g, 12 calories

4 cups apples, peeled, cored and cut into ¼-inch (½ cm) slices, about 480 g, 264 calories

For the streusel topping, combine the flour, sugar, baking powder, and cinnamon in a small bowl. Cut the butter into small pieces and blend into the flour mixture with a pastry blender or a spoon to form crumbs. Refrigerate at least thirty minutes before using.

Preheat oven to 350°F (175°C).
Line standard muffin tin with baking cups and spray with nonstick spray.
Puree the applesauce in a blender or a food processor (the applesauce needs to be finely pureed and smooth) and then measure 1 cup.
Sift the flour, baking powder, and baking soda into a large bowl. Mix in the sugar and the cinnamon.
In another large bowl, whisk together eggs, yogurt, applesauce, lemon zest, salt, and vanilla.
Add the wet ingredients to the dry ingredients, and fold in the apples. Stir just to combine (do not over-mix or you will have tough muffins).
Use an ice cream scoop to distribute the batter evenly among the baking cups, filling each three-quarters full, then sprinkle the streusel topping evenly.

Bake for approximately twenty-five to thirty minutes or until a toothpick tests clean or with a few crumbs (do not over-bake or you will have dry muffins). Cool in the pan for a few minutes before removing to a cooling rack. Muffins can be stored up to two days at room temperature in airtight containers.

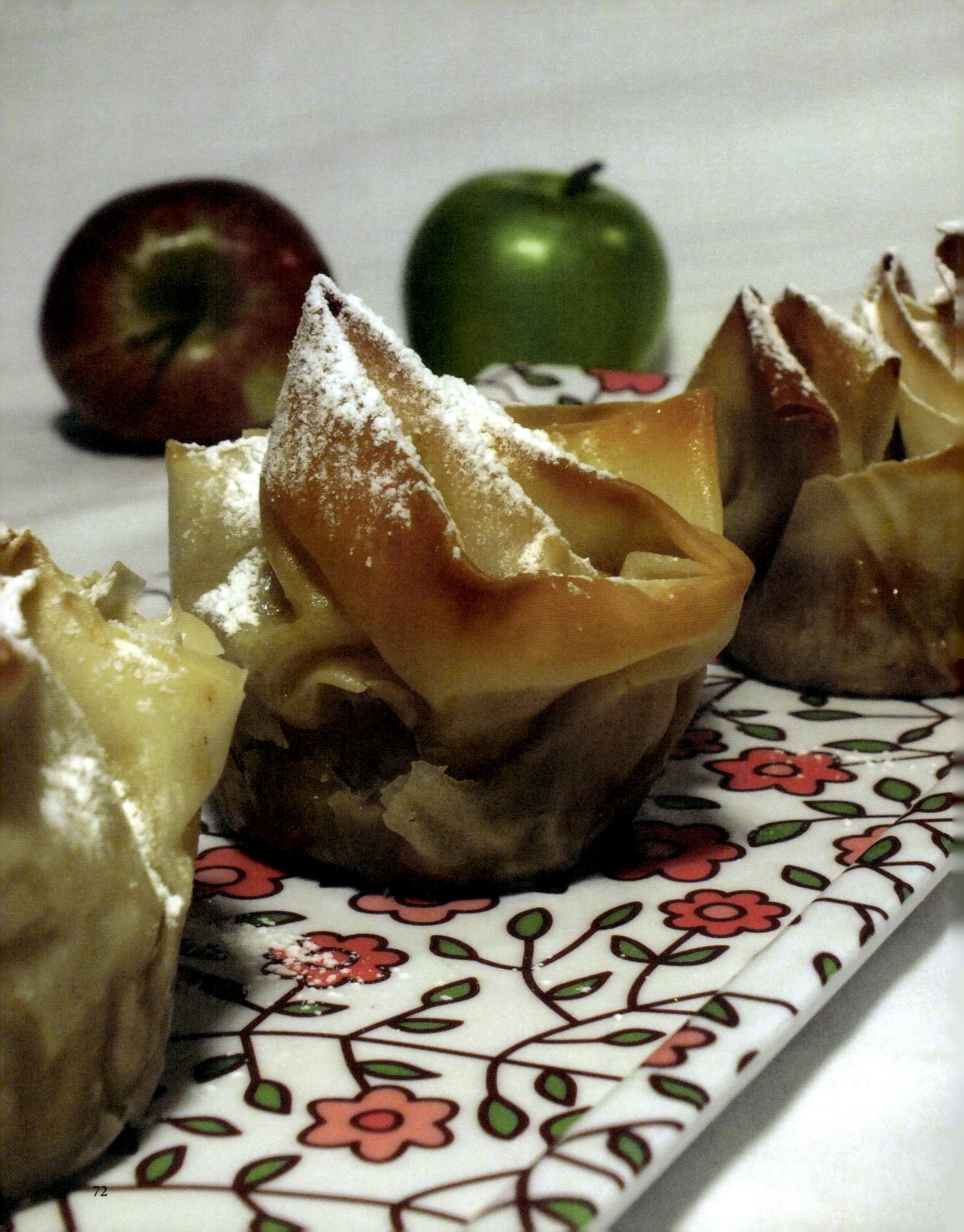

Apple Strudel
Yield: 12 strudels | Per serving: 1 strudel – 143 calories

7 cups apples, peeled, cored and cut into ¼-inch (½ cm) slices, about 840 g, 462 calories

1¼ cups light brown sugar (not firmly packed), 150 g, 562 calories

2 tablespoons unsalted butter, 28 g, 200 calories

1½ teaspoons ground cinnamon, 3 g, 9 calories

1½ teaspoons cornstarch (corn flour), 4 g, 15 calories

1 tablespoon water

Butter-flavored nonstick baking spray, 50 calories

12 sheets of phyllo (fillo) pastry. Sheet size 9"x14" (22x35 cm) is preferable (I used Athens brand), though you can cut other sizes, 132 g, 384 calories

1 tablespoon powdered (confectioners') sugar, 8 g, 32 calories

In a large nonstick skillet or griddle over medium-high heat, add the apples, light brown sugar, butter, and cinnamon. Sauté until the apples begin to soften, approximately ten minutes. Meanwhile, combine cornstarch and 1 tablespoon water in a small glass and add to the apples in the last two minutes of cooking. Make sure there are no liquids left in the skillet. Set the cooked apples aside and let them cool completely.

Preheat oven to 350°F (175°C).
Line a standard muffin tin with paper liners (or baking cups) and spray with nonstick baking spray.
Open the phyllo pastry sheets and layer 1 phyllo sheet, lightly coating with butter-flavored nonstick baking spray. Make sure to keep the unbuttered phyllo covered with a damp towel.
To prevent edges from cracking, spray edges first and then work into center. Fold the sheet in half and spray again. Fold it again; the sheet is now one-quarter of its original size.

Place into the muffin cup. Carefully push phyllo into cup, pressing firmly against bottom and sides (do not worry if the phyllo tears a little bit). Repeat eleven times to make twelve shells. Spoon apple mixture into phyllo and gather points to close the phyllo. Spray again. Bake until golden brown, ten to twenty minutes.
To finish, dust with powdered (confectioners') sugar just before serving.
Best served warm.

Note:
There are two important things about phyllo: 1) Get everything ready before opening the packet of pastry; once the phyllo is open, it will dry quickly; 2) Cover phyllo completely with plastic wrap, then a damp towel.

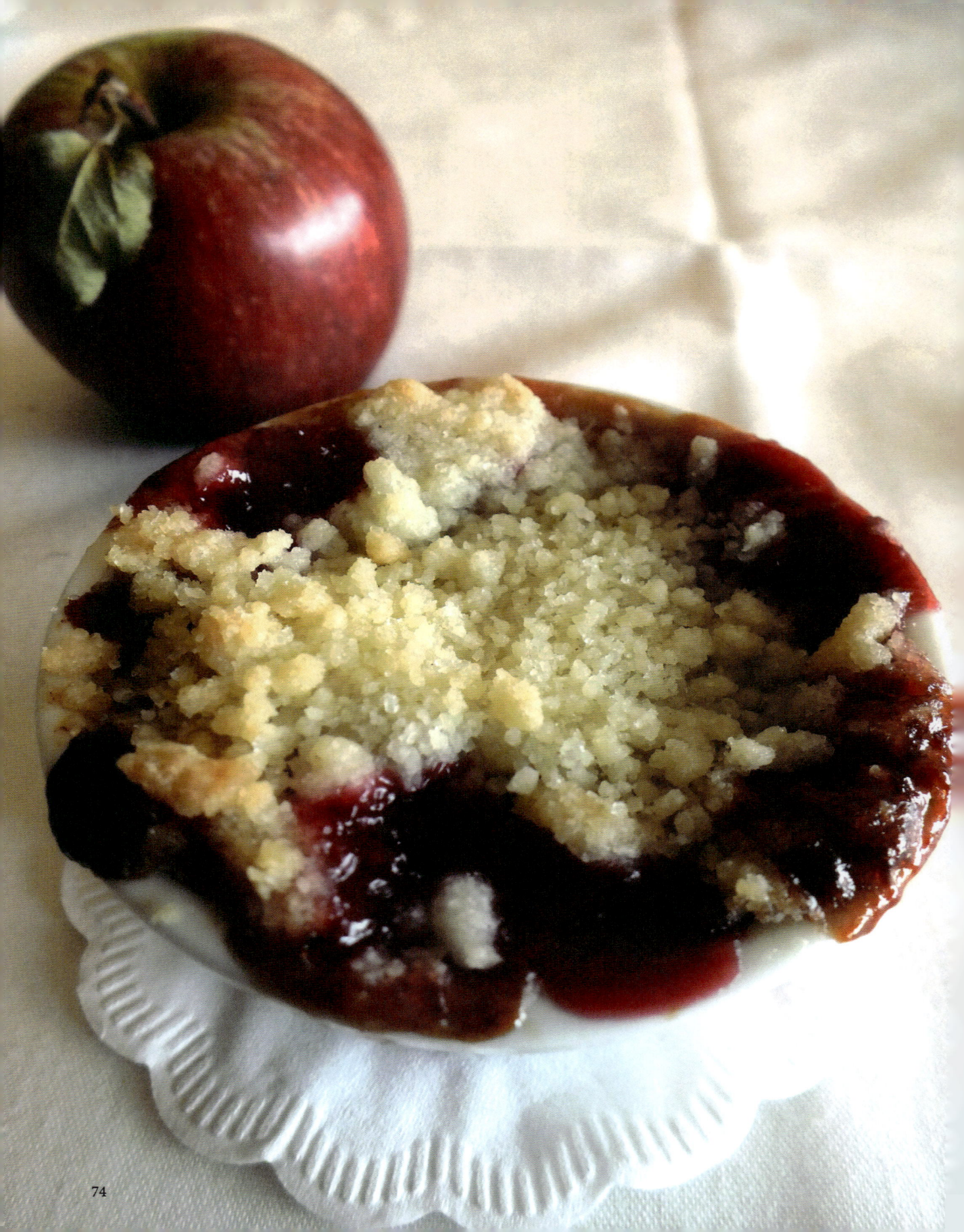

Seasonal Crumble
Yield: 6 crumbles | Per serving: 1 crumble – 159 calories

For the topping:

6 tablespoons all-purpose flour, 48 g, 162 calories

6 tablespoons granulated sugar, 72 g, 270 calories

¼ teaspoon baking powder

3 tablespoons unsalted butter, 42 g, 300 calories

For the crumble:

1 tablespoon granulated sugar, 12 g, 45 calories

1½ teaspoons cornstarch (corn flour), 4 g, 15 calories

2 cups fruit salad made from your favorite fresh fruit chopped into ½-inch (1 cm) chunks (plums, apples, blueberries, cherries, peaches, and raspberries are all very nice), 280 g, 160 calories

Special equipment: Six 2.5- to 3-ounce (80ml) ramekins

Start with the topping: combine the flour, sugar, and baking powder in a small bowl. Cut the butter into small pieces and blend into the flour mixture with a pastry blender or two knives or a spoon to form crumbs. Refrigerate at least thirty minutes before using.

Preheat oven to 350°F (175°C).
In a medium mixing bowl, combine 1 tablespoon sugar and the cornstarch. Add the fruit salad and combine. Transfer evenly to six ramekins. Spread the topping evenly over the fruit. Bake for about forty minutes, or until the topping is browned and the fruit juices are bubbling. Serve immediately. Refrigerate leftovers and reheat before serving.

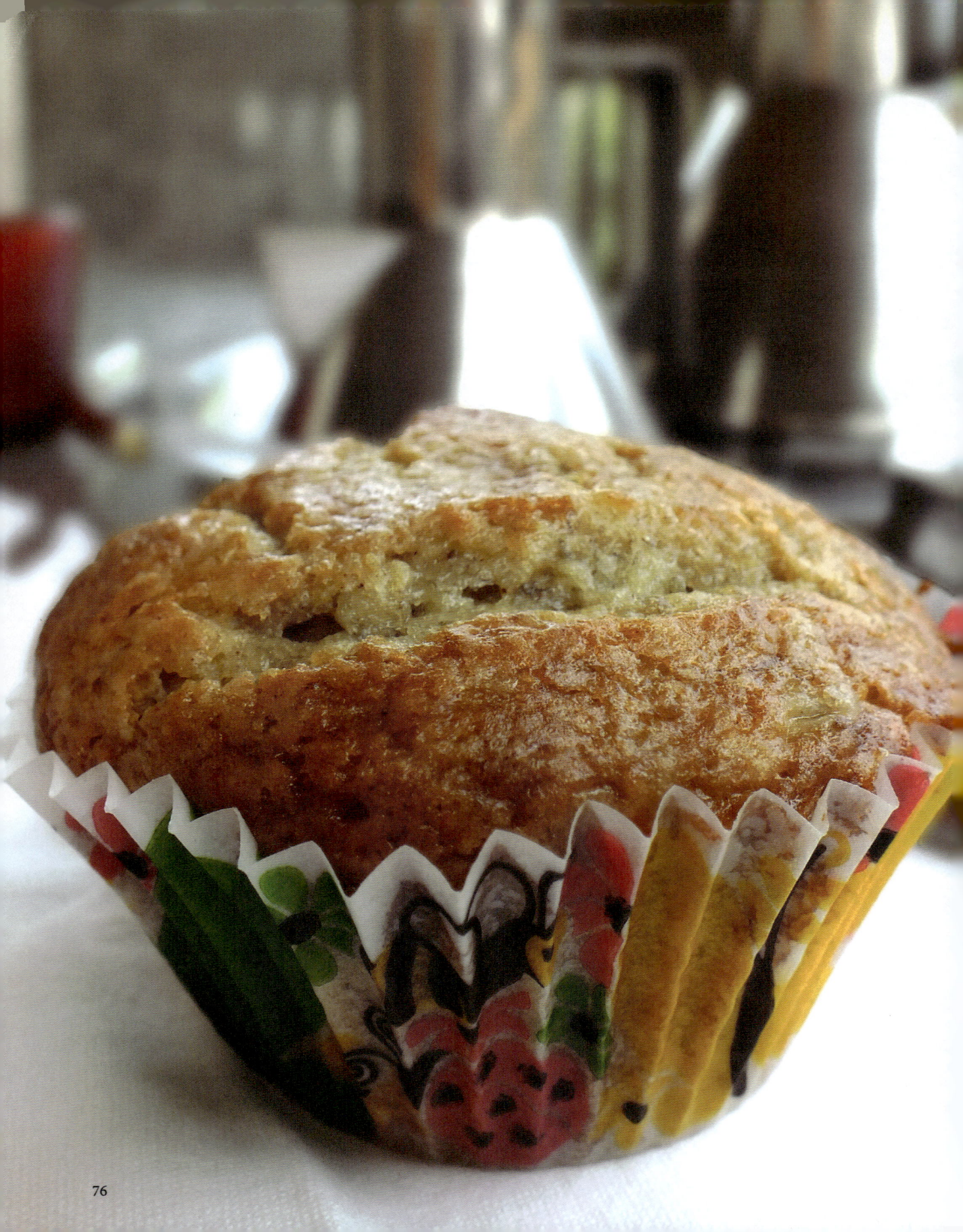

Banana-Cinnamon Muffins
Yield: 17 muffins | Per serving: 1 muffin – 155 calories

2 cups all-purpose flour, 260 g,
866 calories

2 teaspoons baking powder

1 teaspoon baking soda

2 teaspoons ground cinnamon, 4 g,
12 calories

1 cup granulated sugar, 200 g,
750 calories

2¼ cups mashed ripe bananas, 500 g,
445 calories

3 tablespoons vegetable oil, 42 g,
372 calories

2 extra-large eggs, 160 calories

¼ cup orange juice, 60 ml, 27 calories

1 teaspoon vanilla extract, 4 g,
12 calories

¼ teaspoon fine salt

Preheat oven to 350°F (175°C).
Line a standard muffin tin with paper liners (or baking cups) and spray with nonstick baking spray.
Put a pan (or any similar baking dish) with 1 cup of water on the bottom rack of the oven.

Sift the flour, baking powder, baking soda, and cinnamon into a medium-sized bowl. Mix in the sugar.
In another medium bowl, puree the bananas with a fork. Whisk in the oil, eggs, orange juice, vanilla, and salt until the mixture is combined and smooth.
Make a well in the flour mixture and pour in the liquid mixture. Stir just to combine (do not over-mix or you will have tough muffins).

Use an ice cream scoop to distribute the batter evenly among the baking cups, filling each 90 percent full. Bake for approximately twenty to twenty-five minutes or until a toothpick tests clean or with few crumbs. Cool in the pan for a few minutes before removing to a cooling rack. Muffins can be stored up to two days at room temperature in airtight containers.

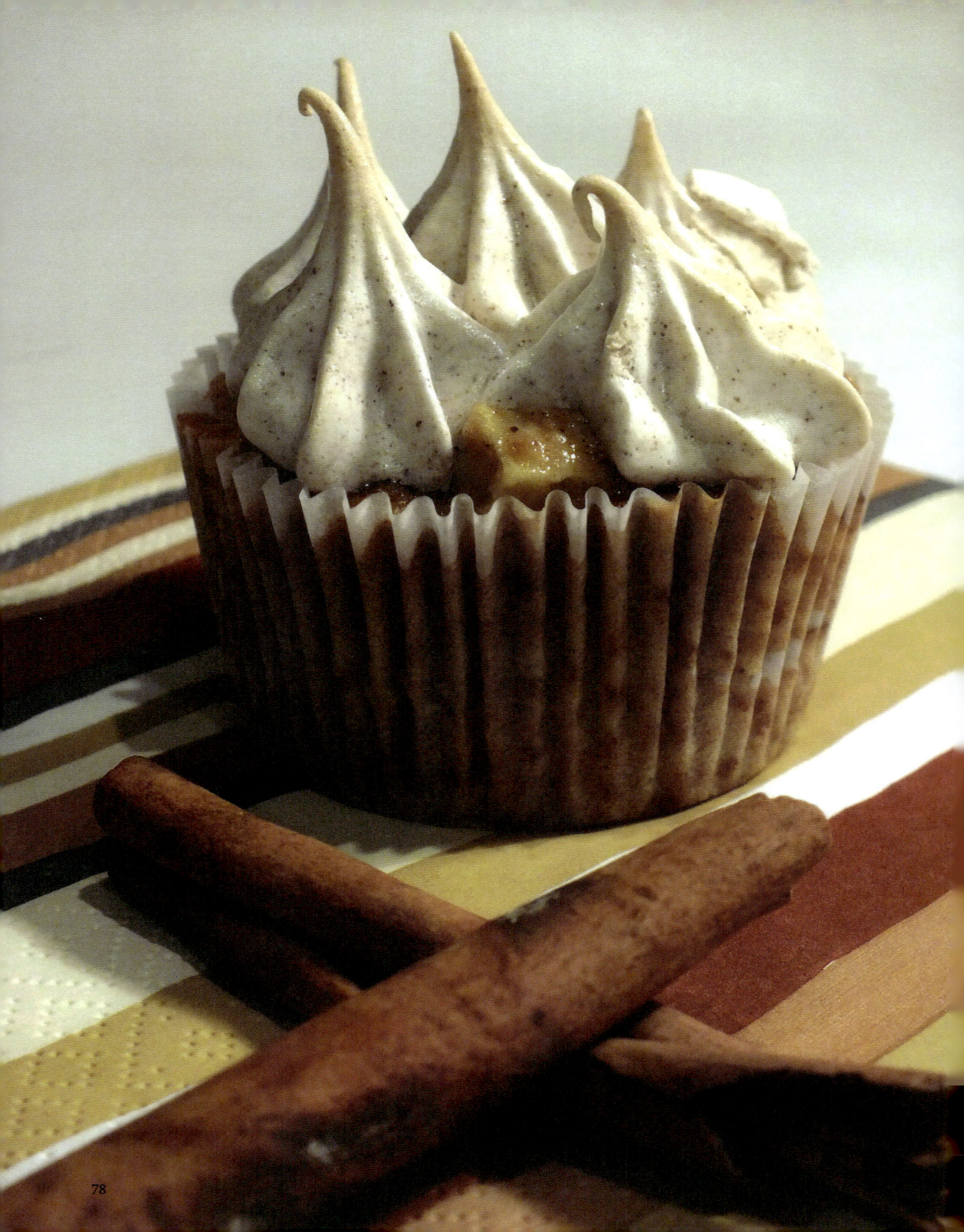

Cinnamon Meringue Apple Cupcakes

Yield: 18 cupcakes | Per serving: 1 cupcake – 144 calories

For the apple cupcakes:

1½ cups all-purpose flour, 195 g, 650 calories

1½ teaspoons baking powder

½ teaspoon baking soda

1 cup granulated sugar, 200 g, 750 calories

2 teaspoons ground cinnamon, 4 g, 12 calories

1 cup unsweetened applesauce, 210 g, 86 calories

1 extra-large egg, 80 calories

3 extra-large egg yolks, 192 calories

¾ cup Greek yogurt 2%, 180 g, 135 calories

½ teaspoon finely grated lemon zest

½ teaspoon fine salt

1 teaspoon vanilla extract, 4 g, 12 calories.

4 cups apples, peeled, cored and cut into ¼-inch (½ cm) slices, about 480 g, 264 calories

For the cinnamon meringue:

2 egg whites at room temperature, 32 calories

¼ teaspoon fine salt

½ cup granulated sugar, 100 g, 375 calories

½ teaspoon vanilla extract, 2 g, 6 calories

¼ teaspoon ground cinnamon

Preheat oven to 350°F (175°C).

Line standard muffin tin with baking cups and spray with nonstick spray.

Sift the flour, baking powder, and baking soda together in a large mixing bowl. Mix in the sugar and the cinnamon. Puree the applesauce in a blender or a food processor (the applesauce needs to be finely pureed and smooth) and then measure 1 cup.

In a medium bowl, whisk the egg, egg yolks, Greek yogurt, lemon zest, applesauce, salt, and vanilla.

Make a well in the flour mixture, and pour in the liquid mixture. Stir just to combine and then fold in the apples (do not over-mix or you will have tough cupcakes).

Use an ice cream scoop to distribute the batter evenly among the baking cups, filling each 80 percent full. Bake for approximately twenty-five minutes until firm and golden but not fully baked.

Make the meringue when the cupcakes are in the oven. With an electric mixer—the bowl and beaters must be clean and free of grease—beat the egg whites on medium-high speed until foamy. Add the salt and continue to beat until they hold soft peaks. Add the sugar, a little at a time, and continue to beat until the meringue holds very stiff peaks. Beat in the vanilla extract. Sift cinnamon over the egg whites and gently fold in until just blended. Transfer meringue to a pastry bag fitted with a small open-star tip.

Remove the cupcakes from the oven and pipe four to six starbursts around the perimeter of the warm cupcakes, then pipe another starburst in the center. Return to the oven and bake, about five minutes. Don't over-bake or you will have dry cupcakes.

Cool in the pan for a few minutes before removing to a cooling rack.

Cupcakes can be refrigerated up to two days in airtight containers.

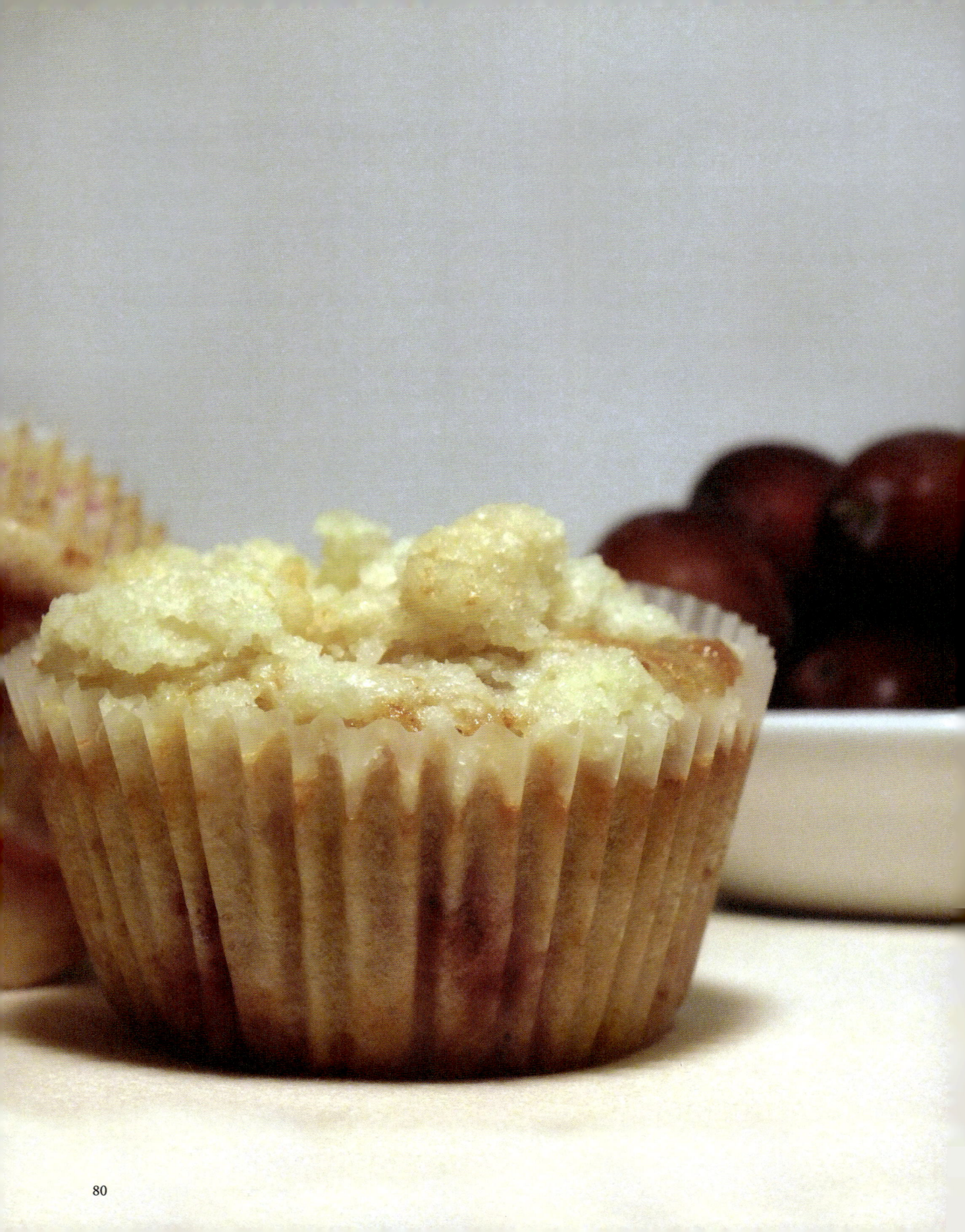

Plum Streusel Muffins

Yield: 14 muffins | Per serving: 1 muffin – 160 calories

For the streusel topping:

2 tablespoons all-purpose flour, 16 g, 54 calories

2 tablespoons granulated sugar, 24 g, 90 calories

¼ teaspoon baking powder

1 tablespoon unsalted butter, 14 g, 100 calories

For the muffins:

1¼ cups all-purpose flour, 163 g, 541 calories

1¼ teaspoons baking powder

¾ cup granulated sugar, 150 g, 562 calories

3 extra-large eggs, 240 calories

¾ cup Greek yogurt 2%, 180 g, 135 calories

2 tablespoons vegetable oil, 28 g, 248 calories

1½ tablespoons honey, 31 g, 96 calories

1 teaspoon vanilla extract, 4 g, 12 calories

¼ teaspoon fine salt

2½ cups fresh plums chopped into bite-sized pieces, 360 g, 155 calories

For the streusel topping, combine the flour, sugar, and baking powder in a small bowl. Cut the butter into small pieces and blend into the flour mixture with a pastry blender or a spoon to form crumbs. Refrigerate at least thirty minutes before using.

Preheat oven to 350°F (175°C).
Line a standard muffin tin with baking cups and spray with nonstick baking spray.
Sift the flour and baking powder into a large bowl. Mix in the sugar.
In another large bowl, whisk together eggs, yogurt, oil, honey, vanilla, and salt.
Make a well in the flour mixture, and pour in the liquid mixture. Stir just to combine and fold in the plums (do not over-mix or you will have tough muffins).
Divide batter evenly among baking cups, filling each 80 percent full, then sprinkle the streusel topping evenly.

Bake for approximately twenty to twenty-five minutes. Cool in the pan for a few minutes before removing to a cooling rack.
Muffins can be stored up to two days at room temperature in airtight containers.

Hazelnuts Almonds Raisins

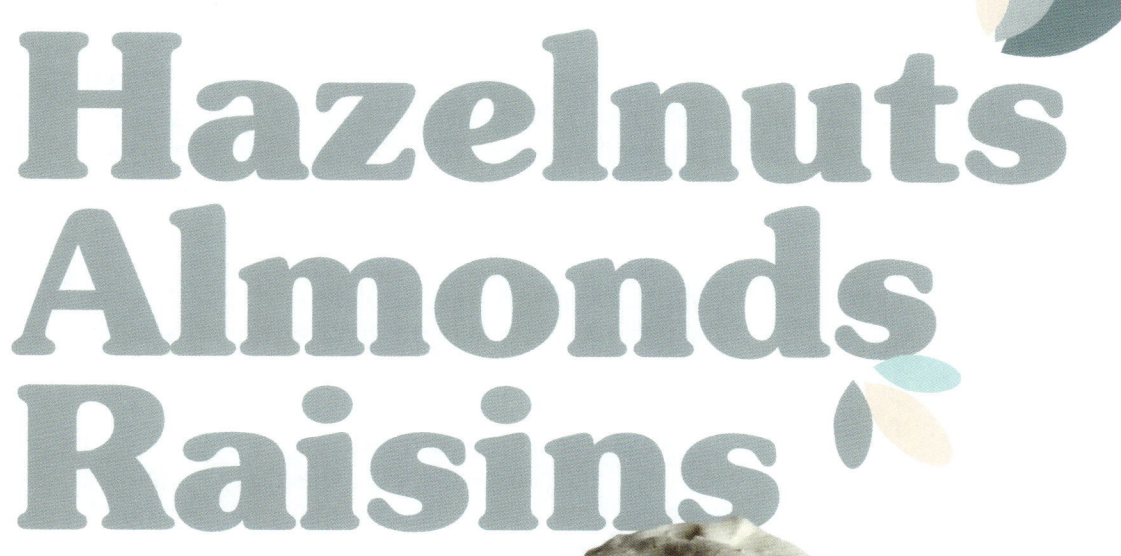
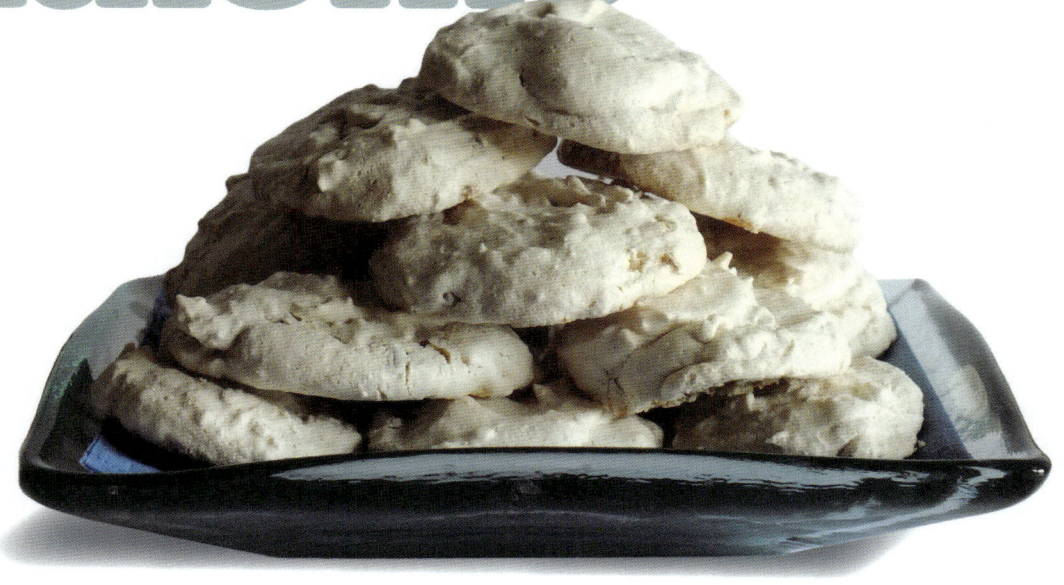

Apple-Raisin Cheese Strudel

Yield: 16 strudels | Per serving: 1 strudel – 144 calories

1 cup Greek yogurt 2%, 240 g, 180 calories

¾ cup ricotta cheese, part skim, 185 g, 257 calories

1 cup granulated sugar, 200 g, 750 calories

2 extra-large eggs, 160 calories

1 teaspoon ground cinnamon, 2 g, 6 calories

1½ teaspoons vanilla extract, 6 g, 18 calories

¼ cup packed raisins (1 small box, 1.5 ounces, 43 g), 129 calories

½ teaspoon fine salt

4 tablespoons all-purpose flour, 32 g, 108 calories

1 cup apples, peeled, cored and cut into ¼-inch (½ cm) slices, about 120 g, 66 calories

Butter-flavored nonstick baking spray, 75 calories

16 sheets of phyllo (fillo) pastry. Sheet size 9"x14" (22x35 cm) is preferable (I used Athens brand), though you can cut other sizes, 182 g, 512 calories

1½ tablespoons powdered (confectioners') sugar, 12 g, 48 calories

Combine the yogurt, cheese, sugar, eggs, cinnamon, vanilla, raisins, and salt in a large bowl. Sift in the flour and then fold in the sliced apples.
Preheat oven to 350°F (175°C).
Line a standard muffin tin with paper liners and spray with nonstick baking spray.

Open the phyllo pastry sheets and layer 1 phyllo sheet, lightly coating with butter-flavored nonstick baking spray. Make sure to keep the unbuttered phyllo covered with a damp towel.
To prevent edges from cracking, spray edges first and then work into center. Fold the sheet in half and spray again. Fold it again; the sheet is now one-quarter of its original size.

Place into the muffin cup. Carefully push phyllo into cup, pressing firmly against bottom and sides (don't worry if the phyllo tears a little bit). Repeat fifteen times to make sixteen shells. Spoon cheese mixture into phyllo and gather points to close the phyllo. Spray again. Bake until golden brown, ten to twenty minutes.
Cool in the pan for a few minutes before removing to a cooling rack.
To finish, dust with powdered (confectioners') sugar just before serving.
Best served at room temperature.

Note:
There are two important things about phyllo: 1) Get everything ready before opening the packet of pastry; once the phyllo is open, it will dry quickly; 2) Cover phyllo completely with plastic wrap, then a damp towel.

Raisin Chocolate Rice Krispies Treats

Yield: 12 treats | Per serving: 1 treat – 137 calories

3¼ cups Rice Krispies, 85 g, 330 calories

½ cup raisins, 70 g, 198 calories

¼ cup of water

8 ounces semi-sweet chocolate, cut into ½-inch chunks (or 1⅓ cups chocolate chips), 224 g, 1,120 calories

Line standard muffin tin with baking cups and spray with nonstick spray.

Put the Rice Krispies and the raisins in a large mixing bowl. Add water to chocolate in a small saucepan over very low heat. Stir until chocolate is melted and mixture is completely smooth. Remove from heat and let cool approximately five minutes. Pour over the Rice Krispies. Mix together quickly using two spoons. Distribute evenly among the baking cups, and press down gently on each. Cover the tin loosely with a plastic bag and freeze at least one hour.

Box them up and keep in the refrigerator for a few days.

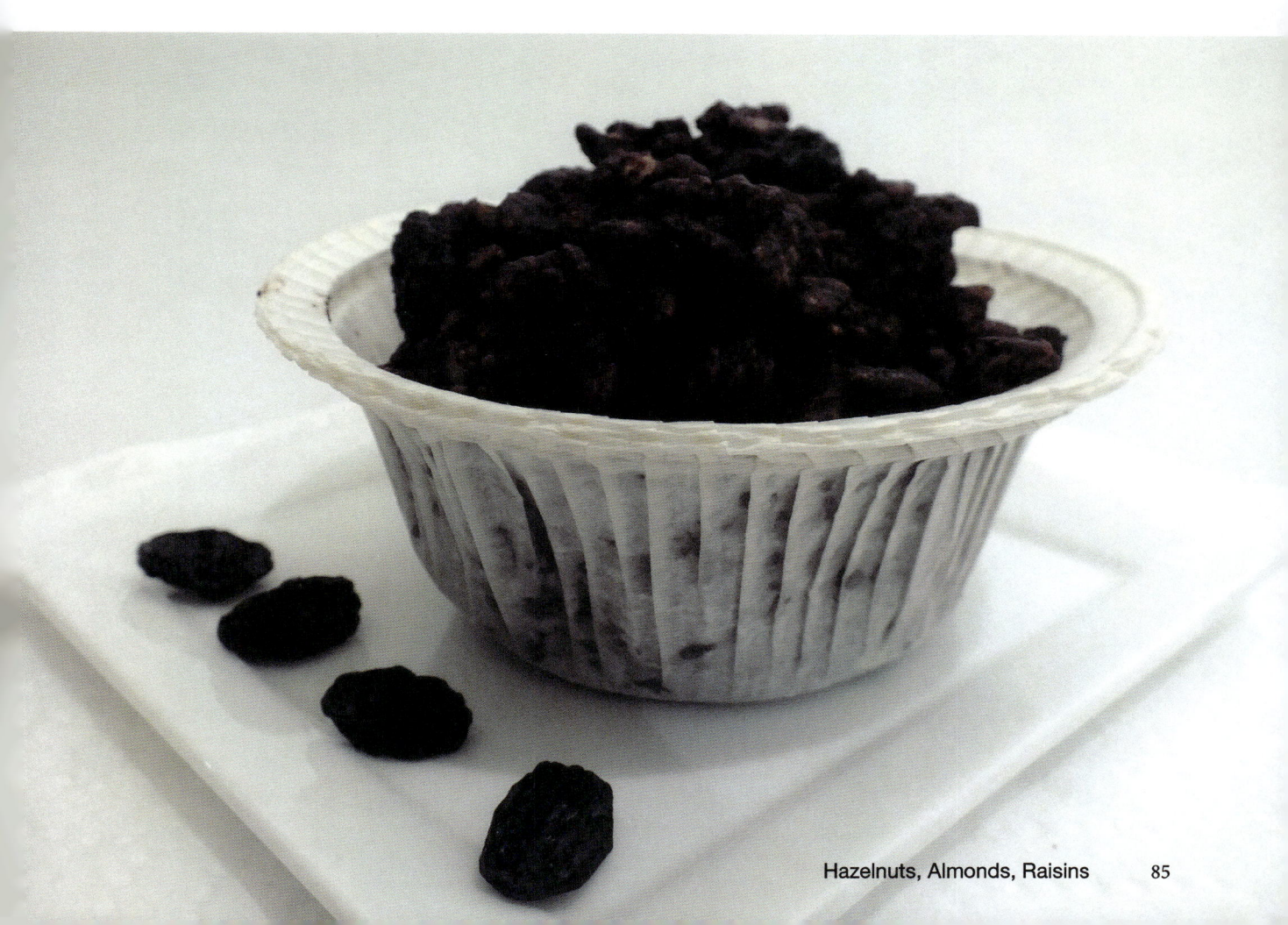

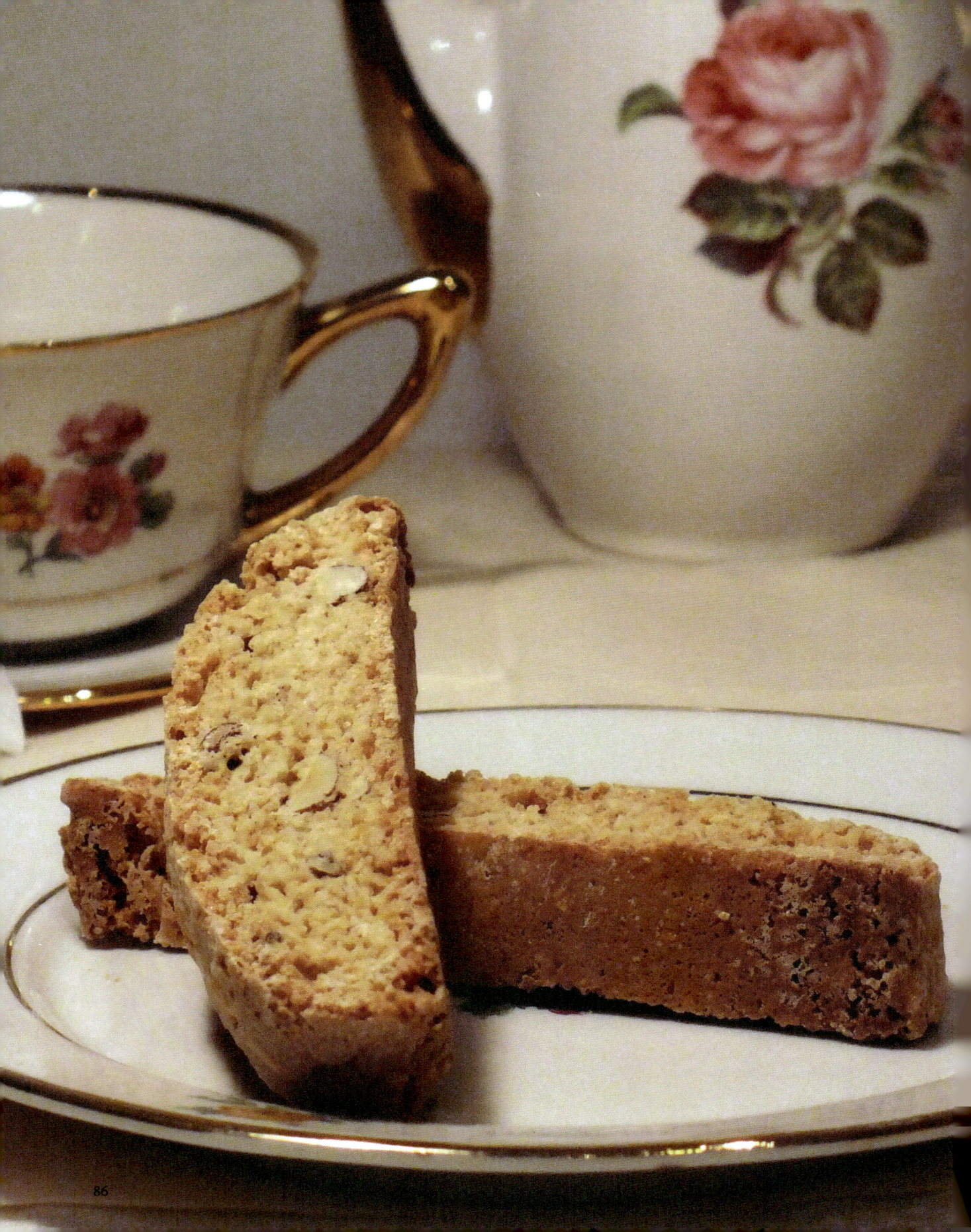

Almond Biscotti

Yield: 40 biscotti | Per serving: 2 biscotti – 154 calories; 1 biscotto – 77 calories

2½ cups all-purpose flour, 325 g, 1,083 calories

2 teaspoons baking powder

1¼ cups granulated sugar, 250 g, 937 calories

¼ teaspoon salt

3 extra-large eggs, 240 calories

1 teaspoon vanilla extract, 4 g, 12 calories

1 cup sliced or coarsely chopped almonds, 140 g, 813 calories

Preheat oven to 350°F (175°C).

Line a baking sheet with parchment paper.

In the bowl of an electric mixer, combine the flour, baking powder, sugar, and salt. In another small bowl, whisk the eggs and vanilla. Gradually add the egg mixture to the flour, and beat until a dough forms, adding almonds about halfway through. If the dough does not form add one to three tablespoons of water.

With floured hands (the dough is quite sticky), divide the dough into two pieces. On a lightly floured surface, roll each half of the dough into a log about sixteen inches (forty centimeters) long and two inches (five centimeters) wide. Transfer the logs to the prepared baking sheet, spacing about four inches (ten centimeters) apart. Logs will spread during baking. Bake until firm to the touch, about twenty-five to thirty minutes. Let cool for about twenty minutes.

Reduce oven temperature to 300°F (150°C).

Cut the logs into slices about ½-inch (1¼ cm) thick using a serrated knife; cut each log into twenty pieces. Arrange the slices, cut side down, on the baking sheet and bake ten minutes, then turn slices over and bake another ten minutes or until golden brown. Remove from oven and let cool on a wire rack.

Cookies can be stored in an airtight container for a month.

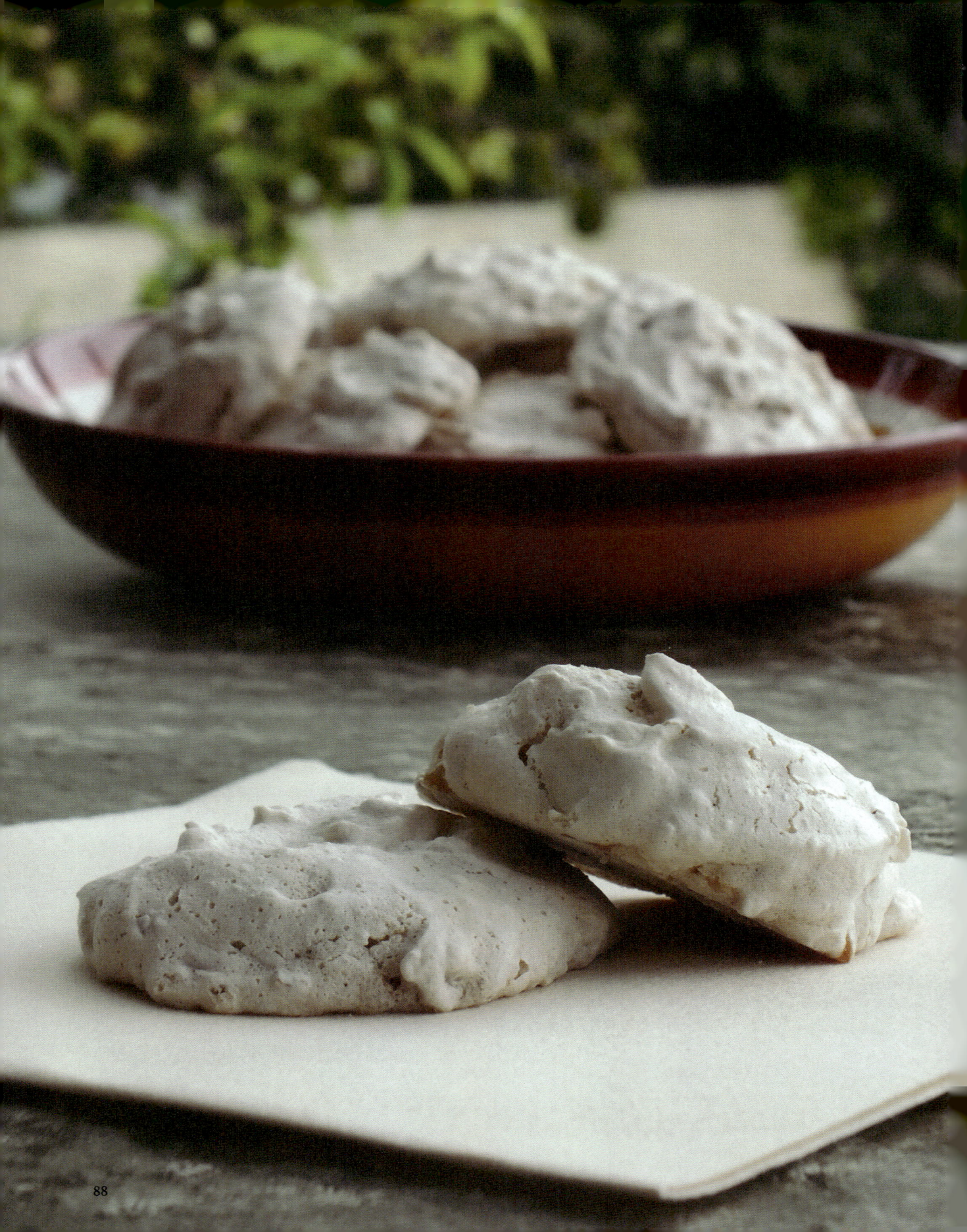

Brutti ma Buoni – Hazelnut

Yield: 20 cookies | Per serving: 2 cookies - 156 calories; 1 cookie - 78 calories

Brutti ma buoni is a delicious Italian cookie that, roughly translated, means, "ugly but good." What I like about them is their delicious nutty-sweet taste and big size.

1 cup chopped hazelnuts, 120 g, 760 calories

2 extra-large egg whites, 32 calories

½ teaspoon salt

1 cup granulated sugar, 200 g, 750 calories

1½ teaspoons vanilla extract, 6 g, 18 calories

Preheat oven to 300°F (150°C).
Line baking sheets with parchment paper, and spray with nonstick baking spray.

Place the hazelnuts on a separate baking sheet and bake for about five minutes or until fragrant. Remove from oven and let cool.
Combine egg whites and salt together in the bowl of an electric mixer—the bowl and beaters must be clean and free of grease—and beat on medium- high speed until soft peaks form (about four minutes). Add the sugar, a little at a time, and continue to beat until the meringue holds very stiff peaks. Beat in the vanilla extract and then fold in the chopped hazelnuts.

Use an ice cream scoop or heaping tablespoonfuls to place dough about two inches apart onto prepared baking sheets. Bake cookies for thirty minutes. Remove from oven and turn the oven to 250°F (120°C). When the oven comes to temperature, place the cookies back in the oven and bake for another thirty minutes. Remove from the oven and let cool to room temperature.
Cookies can be stored up to two days at room temperature in airtight containers.

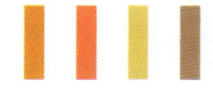

Cheese

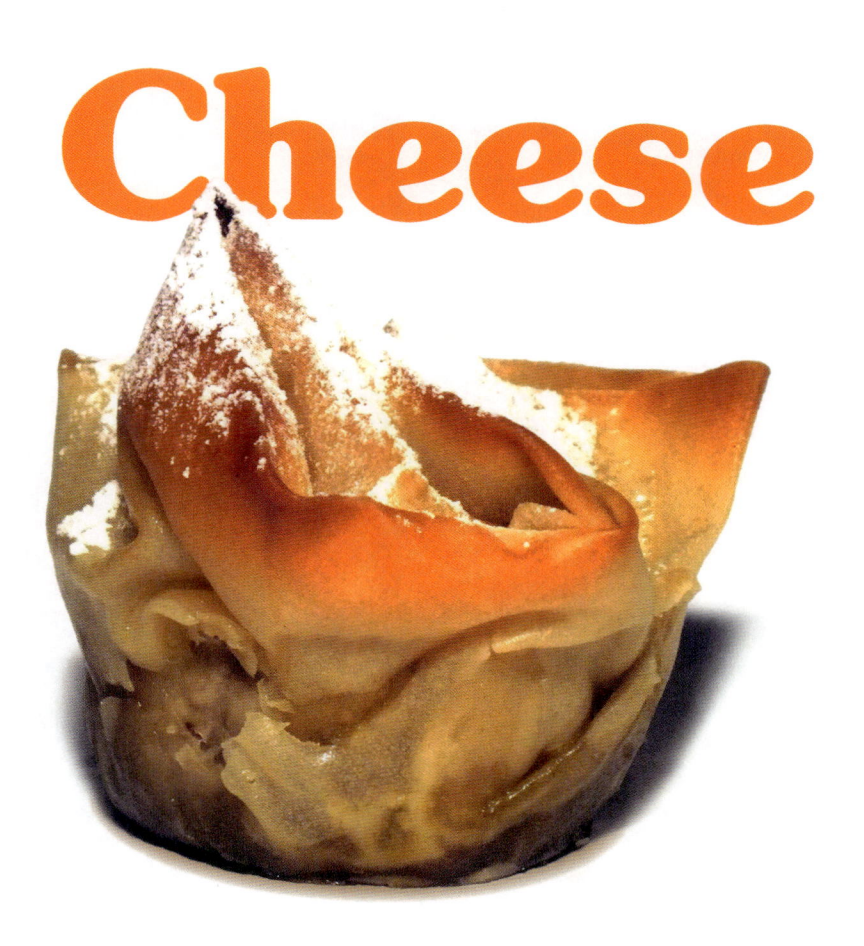

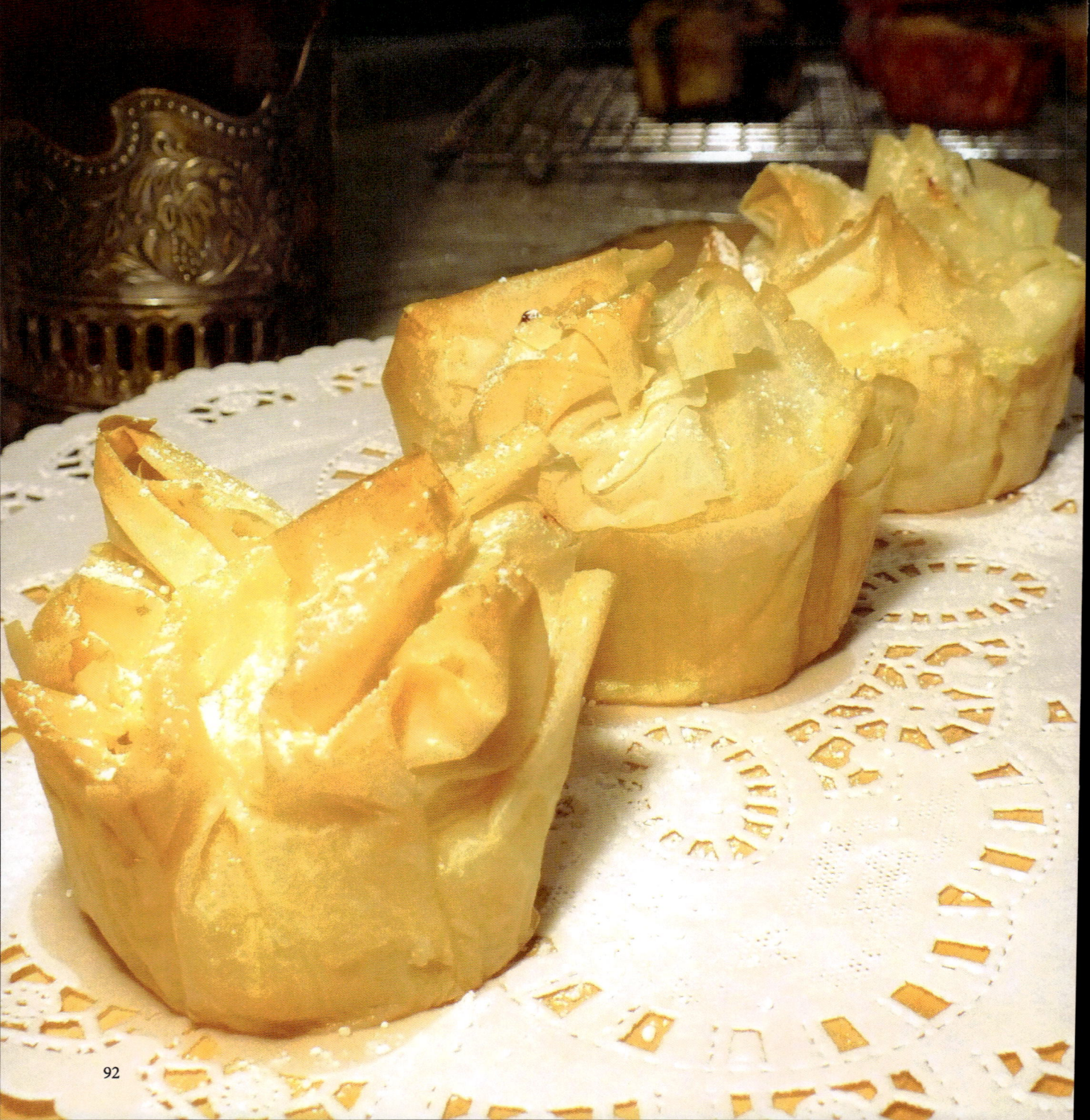

Sweet Cheese Strudel

Yield: 12 strudels | Per Serving: 1 strudel – 149 calories

1 cup Greek yogurt 2%, 240 g, 180 calories

¾ cup ricotta cheese, part-skim, 185 g, 257 calories

¾ cup granulated sugar, 150 g, 562 calories

2 extra-large eggs, 160 calories

¾ teaspoon finely grated lemon zest

1½ teaspoons vanilla extract, 6 g, 18 calories

½ teaspoon fine salt

4 tablespoons all-purpose flour, 32 g, 108 calories

Butter-flavored nonstick baking spray, 50 calories

12 sheets of phyllo (fillo) pastry. Sheet sizes 9"x14" (22x35 cm) is preferable (I used Athens brand), though you can cut other sizes, 132 g, 384 calories

2 tablespoons powdered (confectioners') sugar, 16 g, 64 calories

Combine the yogurt, cheese, sugar, eggs, lemon zest, vanilla, and salt in a large bowl. Sift in the flour and combine.

Preheat oven to 350°F (175°C).
Line a standard muffin tin with paper liners (or baking cups) and spray with nonstick baking spray.
Open the phyllo pastry sheets and layer 1 phyllo sheet, lightly coating with butter-flavored nonstick baking spray. Make sure to keep the unbuttered phyllo covered with a damp towel.
To prevent edges from cracking, spray edges first and then work into center. Fold the sheet in half and spray again. Fold it again; the sheet is now one-quarter of its original size.

Place into the muffin cup. Carefully push phyllo into cup, pressing firmly against bottom and sides (do not worry if the phyllo tears a little bit). Repeat eleven times to make twelve shells. Spoon cheese mixture into phyllo and gather points to close the phyllo. Spray again. Bake until golden brown, ten to twenty minutes.
Cool in the pan for a few minutes before removing to a cooling rack.
Best served at room temperature.
To finish, dust with powdered (confectioners') sugar just before serving.

Note:
There are two important things about phyllo: 1) Get everything ready before opening the packet of pastry; once the phyllo is open, it will dry quickly; 2) Cover phyllo completely with plastic wrap, then a damp towel.

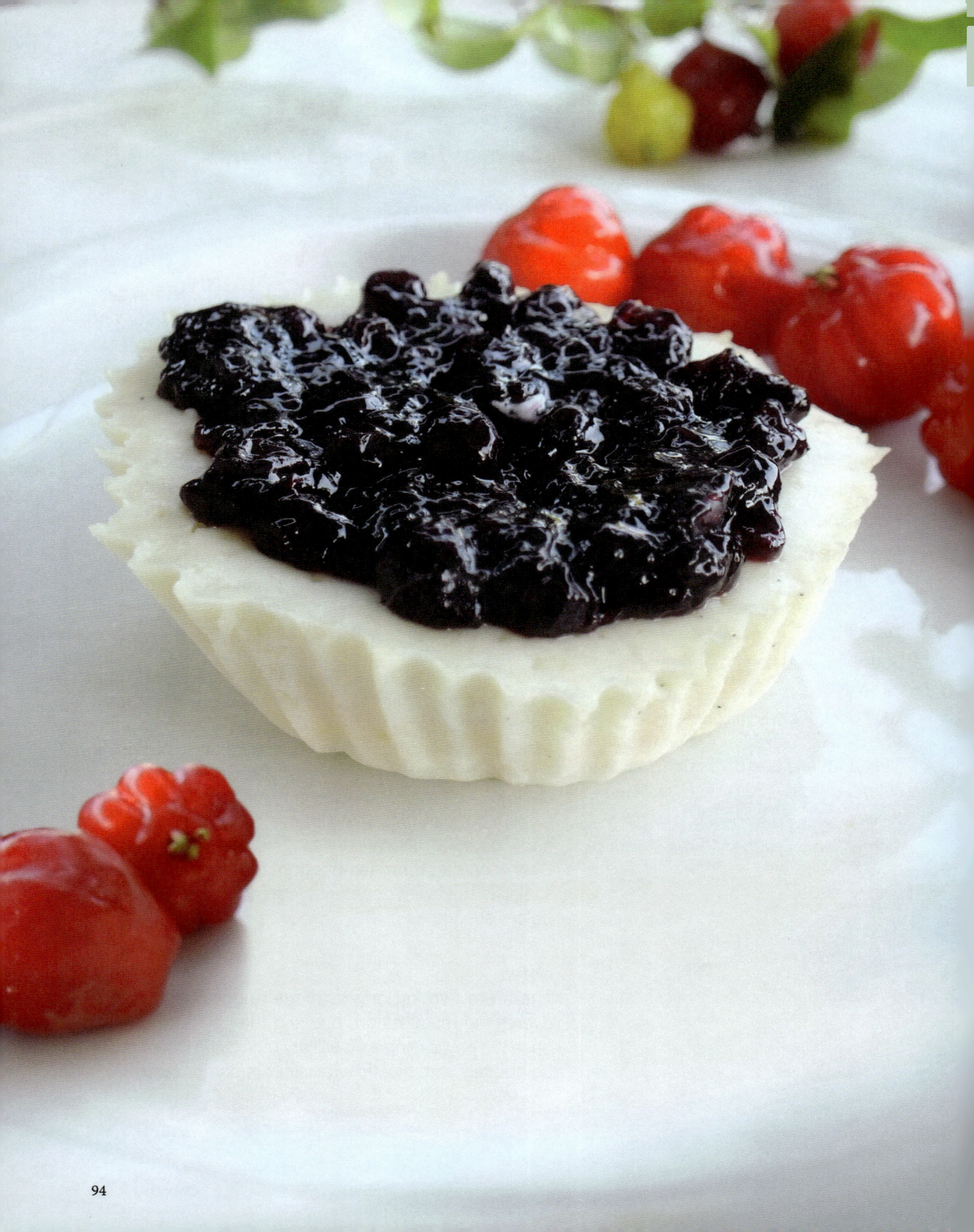

Blueberry Jam Cheese Cupcakes
Yield: 17 cupcakes | Per serving: 1 cupcake – 145 calories

For the cupcakes:

1¾ cups ricotta cheese, part-skim, 425 g, 600 calories

¾ cup Greek yogurt 2%, 180 g, 135 calories

¾ cup light sour cream, 180 g, 234 calories

4 extra-large eggs, 320 calories

1 cup granulated sugar, 200 g, 750 calories

¾ teaspoon finely grated lemon zest

½ teaspoon fine salt

1 tablespoon vanilla extract, 13 g, 37 calories

2 tablespoons all-purpose flour, 16 g, 54 calories

1 tablespoon cornstarch (corn flour) 8 g, 30 calories

For the topping:

17 teaspoons blueberry jam (or your favorite jam), 120 g, 300 calories

Preheat oven to 300°F (150°C).

Line a standard muffin tin with paper liners (or baking cups) and spray with nonstick baking spray.

Put a pan (or any similar baking dish) with 1 cup of hot water on the bottom rack of the oven.

Combine the cheese, yogurt, sour cream, eggs, sugar, lemon zest, salt, and vanilla in a large bowl. Sift the flour and the cornstarch, and combine.

Use an ice cream scoop to distribute the batter evenly among the baking cups, filling each 90 percent full. Bake for approximately one hour and fifteen minutes. Cool in the pan for a few minutes before removing to a cooling rack. Refrigerate at least four hours.

Jam topping: Just before serving, spoon 1 teaspoon jam over each cupcake.

The cupcakes can be refrigerated up to three days in airtight containers.

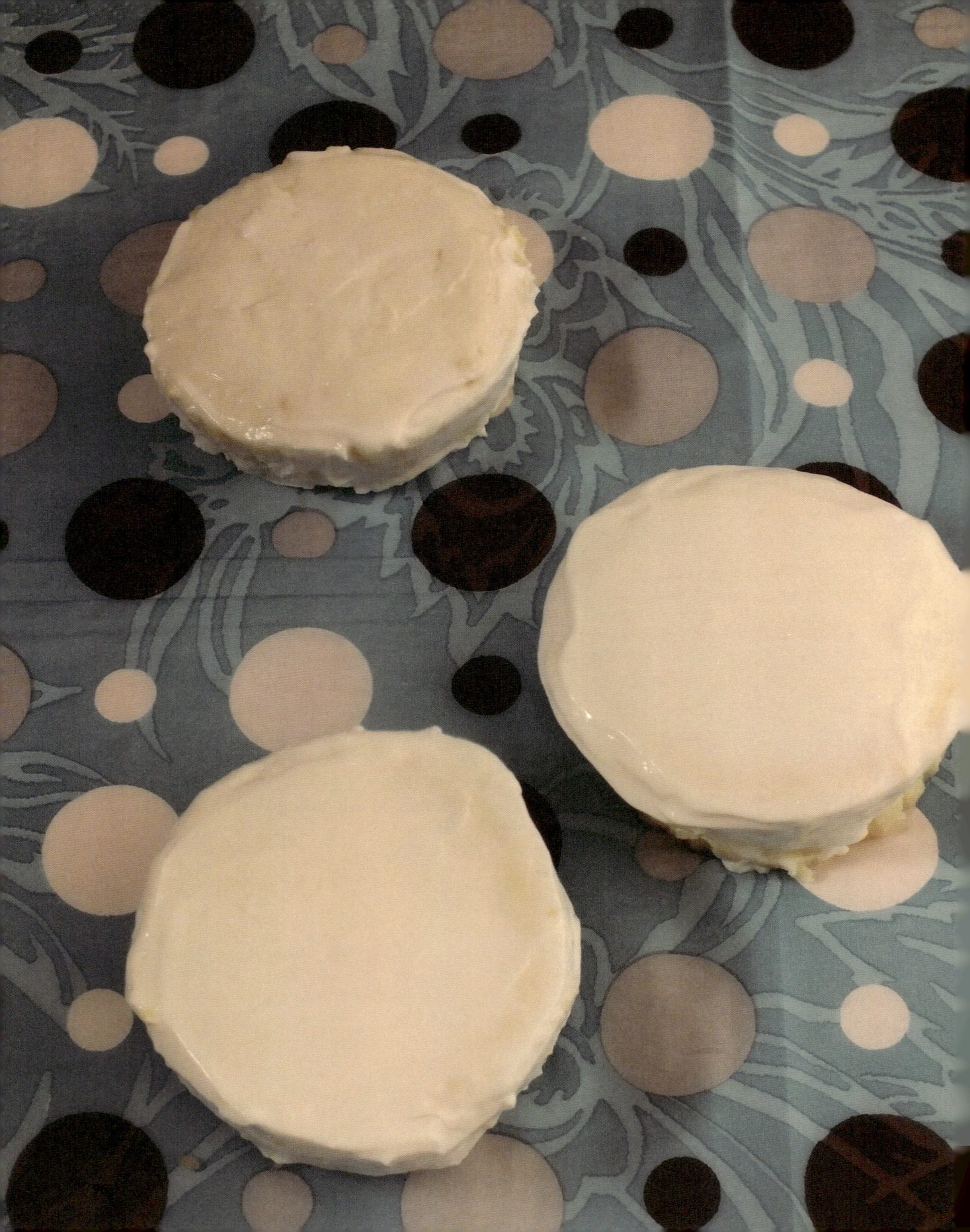

Cheese Cupcakes

Yield: 17 cupcakes | Per serving: 1 cupcake – 152 calories

For the cupcakes:

1¾ cups ricotta cheese, part-skim, 425 g, 600 calories

¾ cup Greek yogurt 2%, 180 g, 135 calories

¾ cup light sour cream, 180 g, 234 calories

4 extra-large eggs, 320 calories

1 cup granulated sugar, 200 g, 750 calories

¾ teaspoon finely grated lemon zest

½ teaspoon fine salt

1 tablespoon vanilla extract, 13 g, 37 calories

2 tablespoons all-purpose flour, 16 g, 54 calories

1 tablespoon cornstarch (corn flour), 8 g, 30 calories

For the topping:

¾ cup sour cream (not low fat), 173 g, 358 calories

1½ tablespoons granulated sugar, 18 g, 67 calories

¼ teaspoon vanilla extract, 3 calories

Preheat oven to 350°F (175°C).
Line a standard muffin tin with paper liners (or baking cups) and spray with nonstick baking spray.
Put a pan (or any similar baking dish) with 1 cup of hot water on the bottom rack of the oven.

Combine the cheese, yogurt, sour cream, eggs, sugar, lemon zest, salt, and vanilla in a large bowl. Sift in the flour and cornstarch, and combine.
Use an ice cream scoop to distribute the batter evenly among the baking cups, filling each 90 percent full. Bake for fifteen minutes and then lower the oven temperature to 250°F (120°C) and continue to bake for about one hour.
Remove from oven and place on a wire rack.
Meanwhile, in a small bowl, combine the sour cream, sugar, and vanilla. Spread the topping over the warm cupcakes and return to oven to bake for fifteen more minutes.

Cool in the pan before removing to a cooling rack.
Refrigerate at least four hours.
Serve cold.
The cupcakes can be refrigerated up to two days in airtight containers.

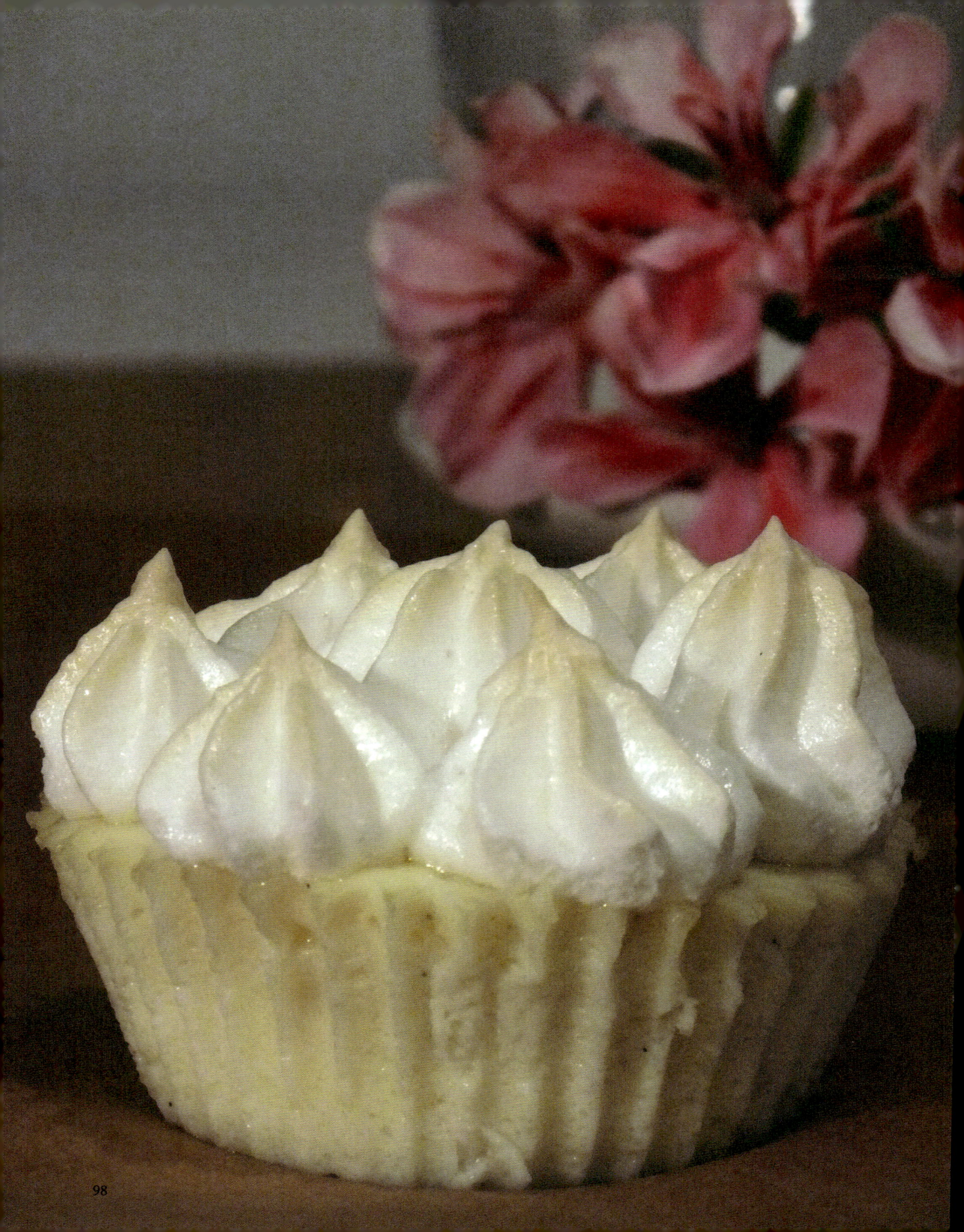

Meringue Cheese Cupcakes

Yield: 17 cupcakes | Per serving: 1 cupcake – 132 calories

For the cupcakes:

1¾ cups ricotta cheese, part-skim, 425 g, 600 calories

¾ cup Greek yogurt 2%, 180 g, 135 calories

¾ cup light sour cream, 180 g, 234 calories

1 extra-large egg, 80 calories

3 egg yolks, 192 calories

½ cup granulated sugar plus 2 tablespoons, 124 g, 465 calories

¾ teaspoon finely grated lemon zest

½ teaspoon fine salt

1 tablespoon vanilla extract, 13 g, 37 calories

2 tablespoons all-purpose flour, 16 g, 54 calories

1 tablespoon cornstarch (corn flour), 8 g, 30 calories

For the meringue:

2 egg whites at room temperature, 32 calories

¼ teaspoon fine salt

½ cup granulated sugar, 100 g, 375 calories

1 teaspoon vanilla extract, 4 g, 12 calories

Preheat oven to 300°F (150°C).

Line a standard muffin tin with paper liners (or baking cups) and spray with nonstick baking spray.

Put a pan (or any similar baking dish) with 1 cup of hot water on the bottom rack of the oven.

Combine the cheese, yogurt, sour cream, egg, egg yolks, sugar, lemon zest, salt, and vanilla in a large mixing bowl. Sift in the flour and cornstarch, and combine.

Use an ice cream scoop to distribute the batter evenly among the baking cups, filling each 90 percent full. Bake for approximately one and a half hours until firm, but not fully baked.

Make the meringue when the cupcakes are in the oven. With an electric mixer—the bowl and beaters must be clean and free of grease—beat the egg whites on medium-high speed until foamy. Add the salt and continue to beat until they hold soft peaks. Add the sugar, a little at a time, and continue to beat until the meringue holds very stiff peaks (about five minutes). Beat in the vanilla extract and scrape down sides of bowl. Transfer meringue to a pastry bag fitted with a small open-star tip.

Remove the cupcakes from the oven and pipe seven starbursts around the perimeter of the cupcakes, then pipe another starburst in the center. Return to the oven and bake about five minutes. Refrigerate at least four hours before serving. Serve cold.

Cupcakes can be refrigerated up to two days in airtight containers

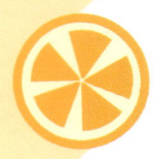

Oranges Lemons Pumpkin

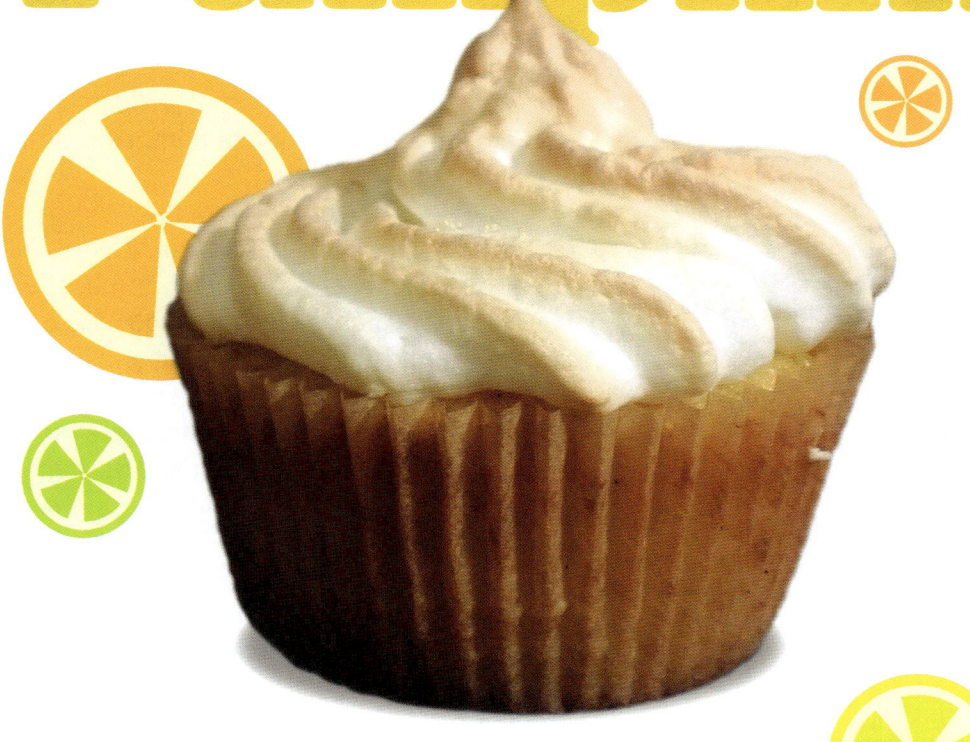

Lemon-Pear Cupcakes

Yield: 18 cupcakes | Per serving: 1 cupcake – 143 calories

For the pear cupcakes:

1½ cups all-purpose flour, 195 g, 650 calories

1½ teaspoons baking powder

½ teaspoon baking soda

1 cup granulated sugar, 200 g, 750 calories

1 cup unsweetened applesauce, 210 g, 86 calories

1 extra-large egg, 80 calories

3 extra-large egg yolks, 192 calories

¾ cup Greek yogurt 2%, 180 g, 135 calories

½ teaspoon fine salt

½ teaspoon finely grated lemon zest

1 teaspoon vanilla extract, 4 g, 12 calories

4 cups ripe pears, peeled, cored and cut into ¼-inch (½ cm) slices, about 450 g, 260 calories

For the lemon meringue:

2 egg whites at room temperature, 32 calories

¼ teaspoon fine salt

½ cup granulated sugar, 100 g, 375 calories

½ teaspoon vanilla extract, 2 g, 6 calories

½ teaspoon finely grated lemon zest

Preheat oven to 350°F (175°C).

Line standard muffin tin with baking cups and spray with nonstick spray.

Sift the flour, baking powder, and baking soda together in a large mixing bowl. Mix in the sugar.

Puree the applesauce in a blender or a food processor (the applesauce needs to be finely pureed and smooth) and then measure 1 cup.

In a medium-sized bowl, whisk the egg, egg yolks, Greek yogurt, applesauce, salt, lemon zest and vanilla.

Add the wet ingredients to the dry ingredients and fold in the pears. Stir just to combine (do not over-mix or you will have tough cupcakes).

Use an ice cream scoop to distribute the batter evenly among the baking cups, filling each 80 percent full. Bake for approximately twenty-five minutes or until firm and golden, but not fully baked.

Make the meringue when the cupcakes are in the oven. With an electric mixer—the bowl and beaters must be clean and free of grease—beat the egg whites on medium-high speed until foamy. Add the salt and continue to beat until they hold soft peaks. Add the sugar, a little at a time, and continue to beat until the meringue holds very stiff peaks. Beat in the vanilla extract and the lemon zest until combined. Transfer meringue to a pastry bag fitted with a small open-star tip.

Remove the cupcakes from the oven and pipe four to six starbursts around the perimeter of the warm cupcakes, then pipe another starburst in the center. Return to the oven and bake about five minutes. Cool in the pan for a few minutes before removing to a cooling rack.

Cupcakes can be refrigerated up to two days in airtight containers.

Double Ginger Muffins

Yield: 17 muffins | Per serving: 1 muffin – 152 calories

2 cups all-purpose flour, 260 g, 866 calories

2 teaspoons baking powder

1 teaspoon baking soda

2 teaspoons cinnamon, 4 g, 12 calories

1 cup granulated sugar, 200 g, 750 calories

3 extra-large eggs, lightly beaten, 240 calories

1 cup canned pumpkin puree (not pie filling), 246 g, 100 calories

1 cup finely grated raw carrots, 125 g, 54 calories

3 tablespoons vegetable oil, 42 g, 372 calories

½ cup orange juice, 120 ml, 54 calories

1 teaspoon vanilla extract, 4 g, 12 calories

¼ teaspoon fine salt

2 tablespoons honey, 42 g, 128 calories

1 teaspoon freshly grated root ginger

½ teaspoon ground ginger

Preheat oven to 350°F (175°C).
Line a standard muffin tin with paper liners (or baking cups) and spray with nonstick baking spray.

Sift the flour, baking powder, baking soda, and the cinnamon into a large bowl. Mix in the sugar.
In another large mixing bowl, whisk the eggs together with the pumpkin puree, carrot, oil, orange juice, vanilla, salt, honey, and ginger until the mixture is combined and smooth.
Make a well in the flour mixture, and pour in the liquid mixture. Stir just to combine (do not over-mix or you will have tough muffins).

Use an ice cream scoop to distribute the batter evenly among the baking cups, filling each 80 percent full. Bake for approximately twenty to twenty-five minutes or until a toothpick tests clean or with a few crumbs. Cool in the pan for a few minutes before removing to a cooling rack. Muffins can be stored up to three days in the refrigerator.

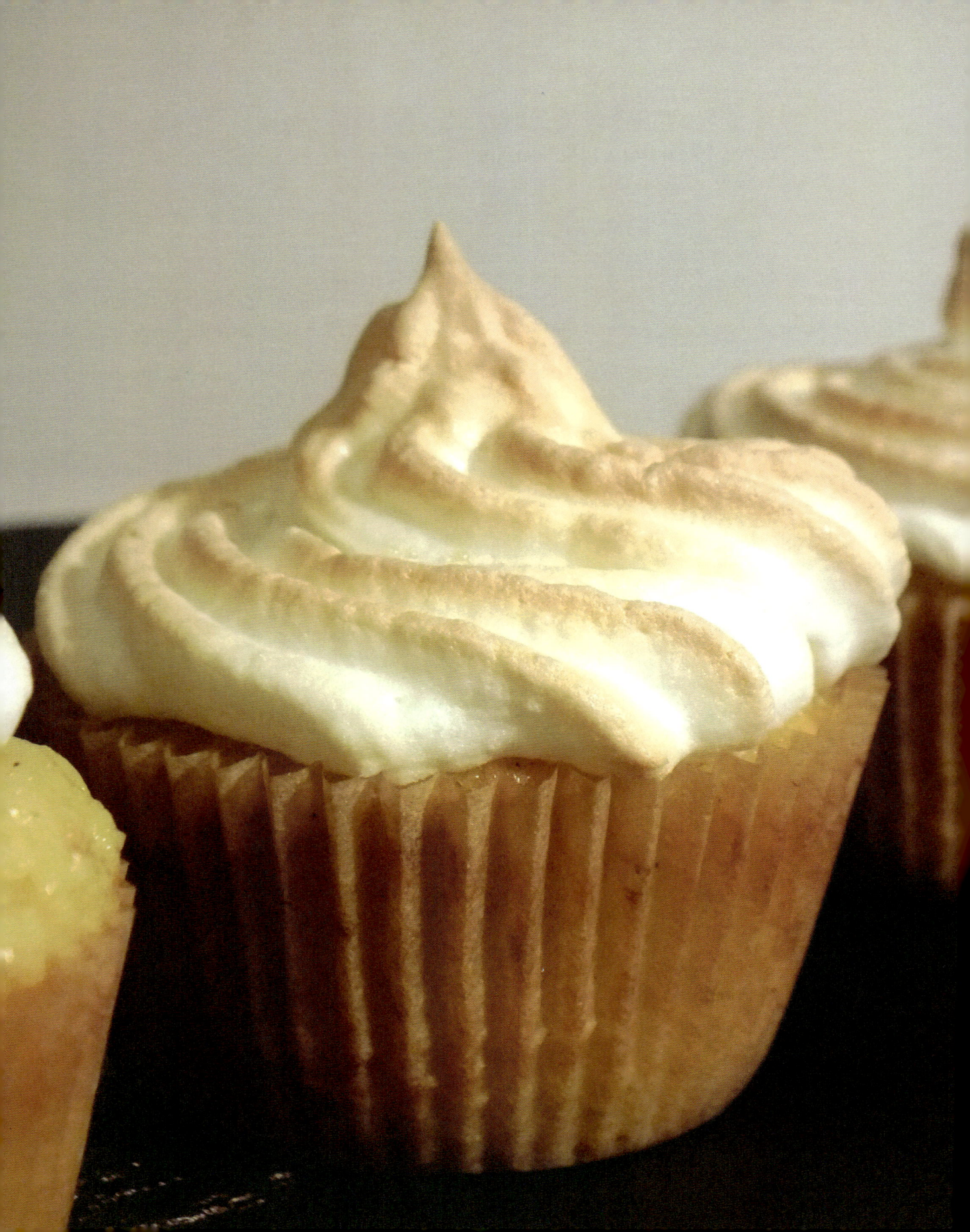

Orange-Lemon Meringue Cupcakes

Yield: 15 cupcakes | Per serving: 1 cupcake – 143 calories

For the cupcakes:

1½ cups all-purpose flour, 195 g, 650 calories

1½ teaspoons baking powder

½ teaspoon baking soda

¾ cup granulated sugar, 150 g, 562 calories

1 cup minus 1 tablespoon Greek yogurt 2%, 225 g, 170 calories

¾ cup orange juice, 180 ml, 81 calories

1 extra-large egg, 80 calories

3 extra-large egg yolks, 192 calories

¼ teaspoon fine salt

For the lemon meringue:

2 egg whites at room temperature, 32 calories

¼ teaspoon fine salt

½ cup granulated sugar, 100 g, 375 calories

½ teaspoon vanilla extract, 2 g, 6 calories

½ teaspoon finely grated lemon zest

Preheat oven to 340°F (170°C).

Line standard muffin tin with baking cups and spray with nonstick spray.

Put a pan (or any similar baking dish) with 1 cup of water on the bottom rack of the oven.

Sift the flour, baking powder, and baking soda together in a large mixing bowl. Mix in the sugar.

In a medium-sized bowl, whisk the Greek yogurt and the orange juice until the mixture is combined and smooth. With an electric mixer, with the whisk attachment, beat the whole egg, 3 egg yolks, and salt on high speed until the batter is thick and fluffy (about two minutes).

Gently fold the yogurt mixture into the eggs until incorporated.

Make a well in the flour mixture, and pour in the liquid mixture. Stir just to combine (do not over-mix or you will have tough cupcakes).

Use an ice cream scoop to distribute the batter evenly among the baking cups, filling each 80 percent full. Bake for approximately twenty minutes until firm but not fully baked.

Make the meringue when the cupcakes are in the oven. With an electric mixer—the bowl and beaters must be clean and free of grease—beat the egg whites on medium-high speed until foamy. Add the salt and continue to beat until they hold soft peaks. Add the sugar, a little at a time, and continue to beat until the meringue holds very stiff peaks. Beat in the vanilla extract and the lemon zest until combined. Transfer meringue to a pastry bag fitted with a large plain tip.

Remove the cupcakes from the oven and pipe a spiral pattern onto each cupcake, starting at the edges and ending with a peak in the center. Return to the oven and bake about five minutes. Don't over-bake or you will have dry cupcakes.

Cool in the pan for a few minutes before removing to a cooling rack.

Cupcakes can be refrigerated up to two days in airtight containers. Bring to room temperature before serving.

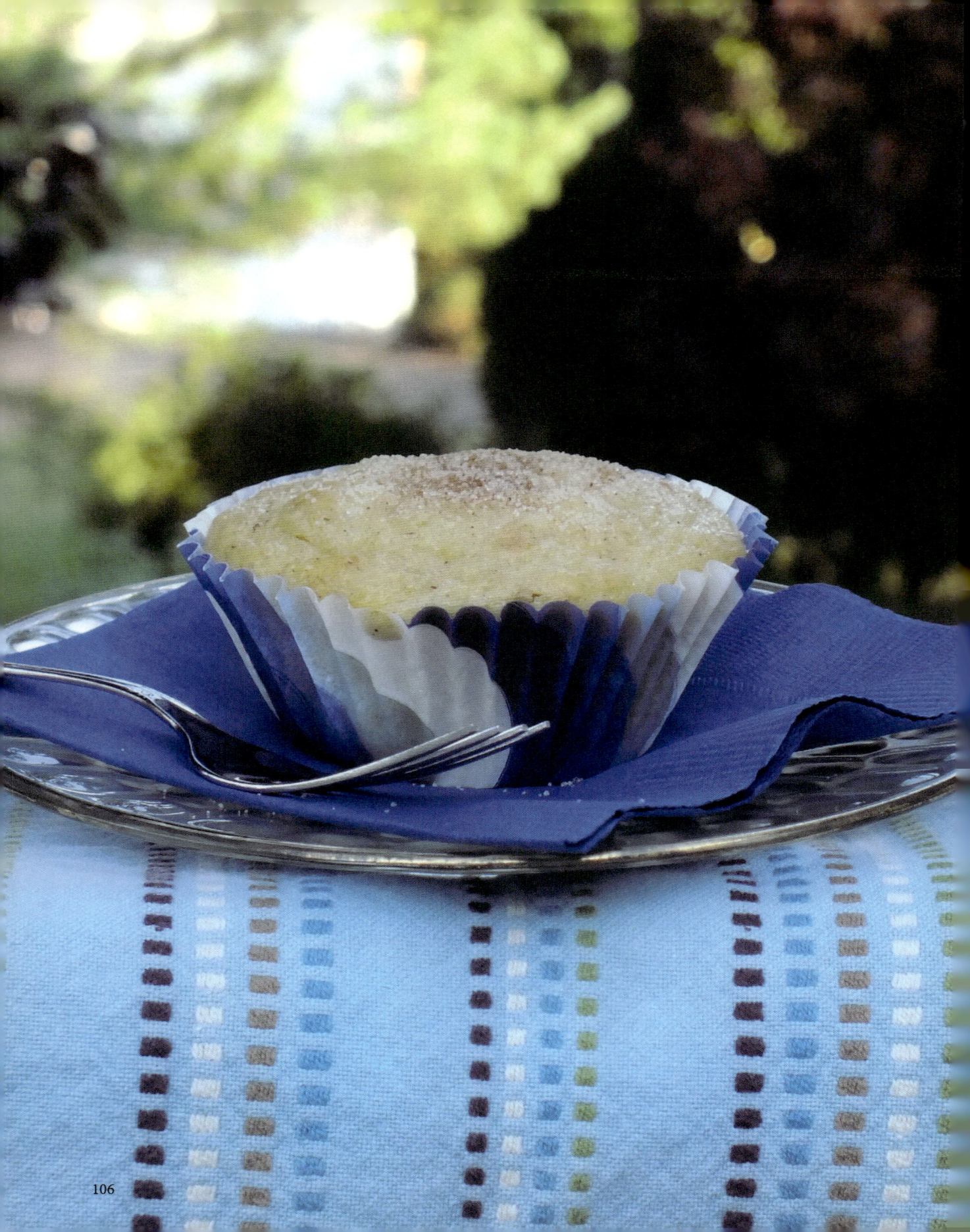

Orange-Cinnamon Muffins

Yield: 15 muffins | Per serving: 1 muffin – 132 calories

For the muffins:

1½ cups all-purpose flour, 195 g, 650 calories

1½ teaspoons baking powder

½ teaspoon baking soda

1 cup granulated sugar, 200 g, 750 calories

1 cup minus 1 tablespoon Greek yogurt 2%, 225 g, 170 calories

¾ cup orange juice, 180 ml, 81 calories

3 extra-large eggs, 240 calories

¼ teaspoon fine salt

For the topping:

2 tablespoons granulated sugar, 24 g, 90 calories

½ teaspoon cinnamon, 1 g, 3 calories

Preheat oven to 340°F (170°C).

Line standard muffin tin with baking cups and spray with nonstick spray.

Put a pan (or any similar baking dish) with 1 cup of water on the bottom rack of the oven.

Sift the flour, baking powder, and baking soda into a large bowl. Mix in the sugar.

In a medium-sized bowl, whisk the Greek yogurt and the orange juice until the mixture is combined and smooth. With an electric mixer, with the whisk attachment, beat the whole eggs together with salt on high speed until they are thick and fluffy (about two minutes). Gently fold the yogurt mixture into the eggs until incorporated.

Make a well in the dry ingredients, and pour in the liquid mixture. Stir just to combine (do not over-mix or you will have tough muffins).

Use an ice cream scoop to distribute the batter evenly among the muffin cups, filling each 90 percent full. Mix the topping ingredients in a small bowl and sprinkle evenly over the muffins.

Bake for approximately twenty to twenty-five minutes or until a toothpick tests clean or with a few crumbs.

Cool in the pan for a few minutes before removing to a cooling rack.

Cakes can be stored up to two days in the refrigerator in airtight containers.

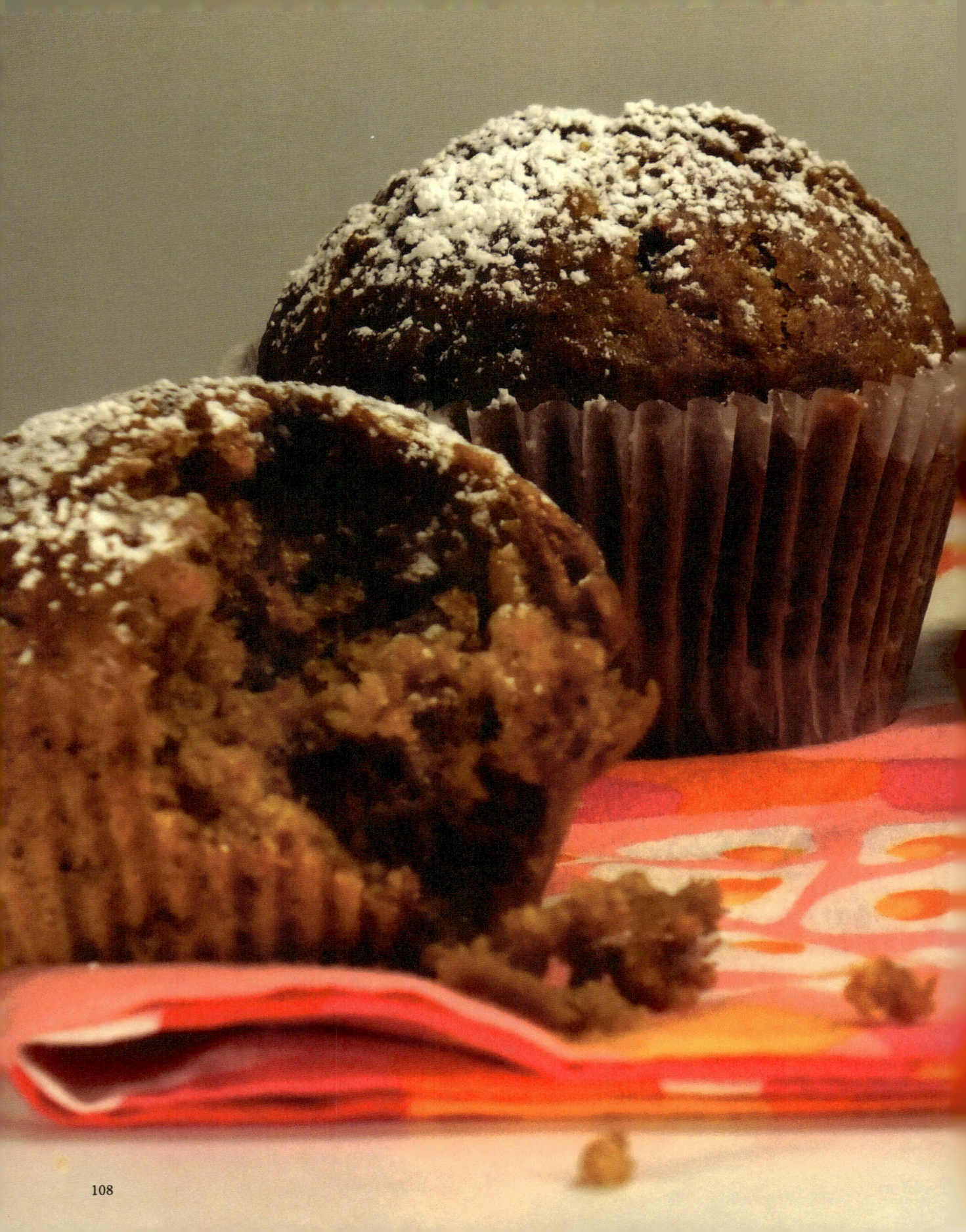

Pumpkin-Cinnamon Muffins
Yield: 17 muffins | Per serving: 1 muffin – 151 calories

2 cups all-purpose flour, 260 g, 866 calories

2 teaspoons baking powder

1 teaspoon baking soda

2 teaspoons cinnamon, 4 g, 12 calories

1 cup granulated sugar, 200 g, 750 calories

⅛ teaspoon grated nutmeg

⅛ teaspoon ground cloves

⅛ teaspoon ground ginger

3 extra-large eggs, lightly beaten, 240 calories

2 cups canned pumpkin puree (not pie filling), 492 g, 200 calories

3 tablespoons vegetable oil, 42 g, 372 calories

¼ cup orange juice, 60 ml, 27 calories

1 teaspoon vanilla extract, 4 g, 12 calories

¼ teaspoon fine salt

3 tablespoons powdered (confectioners') sugar, 24 g, 96 calories

Preheat oven to 350°F (175°C).

Line a standard muffin tin with paper liners (or baking cups) and spray with nonstick baking spray.

Sift the flour, baking powder, baking soda, and cinnamon into a large bowl. Mix in the sugar, nutmeg, cloves, and ginger.

In another large mixing bowl, whisk the eggs together with the pumpkin puree, oil, orange juice, vanilla, and salt until the mixture is combined and smooth.

Make a well in the flour mixture, and pour in the liquid mixture. Stir just to combine (don't over-mix or you will have tough muffins).

Use an ice cream scoop to distribute the batter evenly among the baking cups, filling each 90 percent full. Bake for approximately twenty to twenty-five minutes or until a toothpick tests clean or with a few crumbs (do not over-bake or you will have dry muffins). Cool in the pan for a few minutes before removing to a cooling rack.

To finish, just before serving, dust with powdered sugar. Muffins can be stored up to two days in the refrigerator.

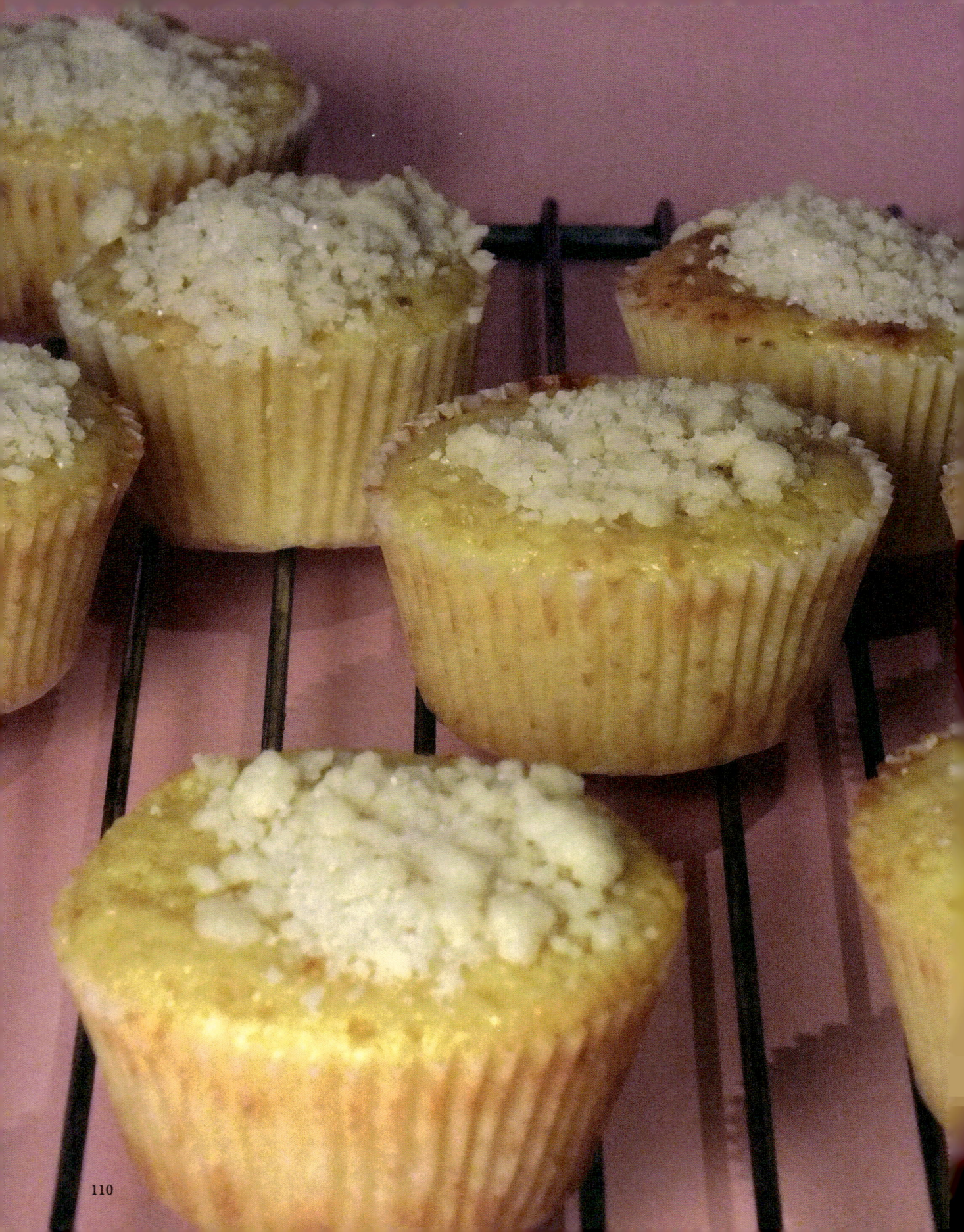

Streusel Orange Muffins
Yield: 15 muffins | Per serving: 1 muffin - 149 calories

For the streusel topping:

3 tablespoons all-purpose flour, 24 g, 81 calories

3 tablespoons granulated sugar, 36 g, 135 calories

¼ teaspoon baking powder

1½ tablespoons unsalted butter, 21 g, 150 calories

For the muffins:

1½ cups all-purpose flour, 195 g, 650 calories

1½ teaspoons baking powder

½ teaspoon baking soda

1 cup granulated sugar, 200 g, 750 calories

1 cup minus 1 tablespoon Greek yogurt 2%, 225 g, 170 calories

½ cup orange juice, 120 ml, 54 calories

3 extra-large eggs, 240 calories

¼ teaspoon fine salt

For the streusel topping, combine the flour, sugar, and baking powder in a small bowl. Cut the butter into small pieces and blend into the flour mixture with a pastry blender or a spoon to form crumbs. Refrigerate at least thirty minutes before using.
Preheat oven to 340°F (170°C).
Line standard muffin tin with baking cups and spray with nonstick spray.

Sift the flour, baking powder, and baking soda into a large bowl. Mix in the sugar.
In a medium-sized bowl, whisk the Greek yogurt and orange juice until the mixture is combined and smooth. With an electric mixer, with the whisk attachment, beat the whole eggs together with salt on high speed until they are thick and fluffy (about two minutes).
Gently fold the yogurt mixture into the eggs until incorporated.
Make a well in the dry ingredients, and pour in the liquid mixture. Stir just to combine (do not over-mix or you will have tough muffins).

Use an ice cream scoop to distribute the batter evenly among the baking cups, filling each 80 percent full. Bake for approximately fifteen minutes until firm, but not fully baked. Remove from oven and sprinkle the streusel topping evenly. Continue baking for another ten minutes. Cool in the pan for a few minutes before removing to a cooling rack.
Muffins can be stored up to two days at room temperature in airtight containers.

Vanilla

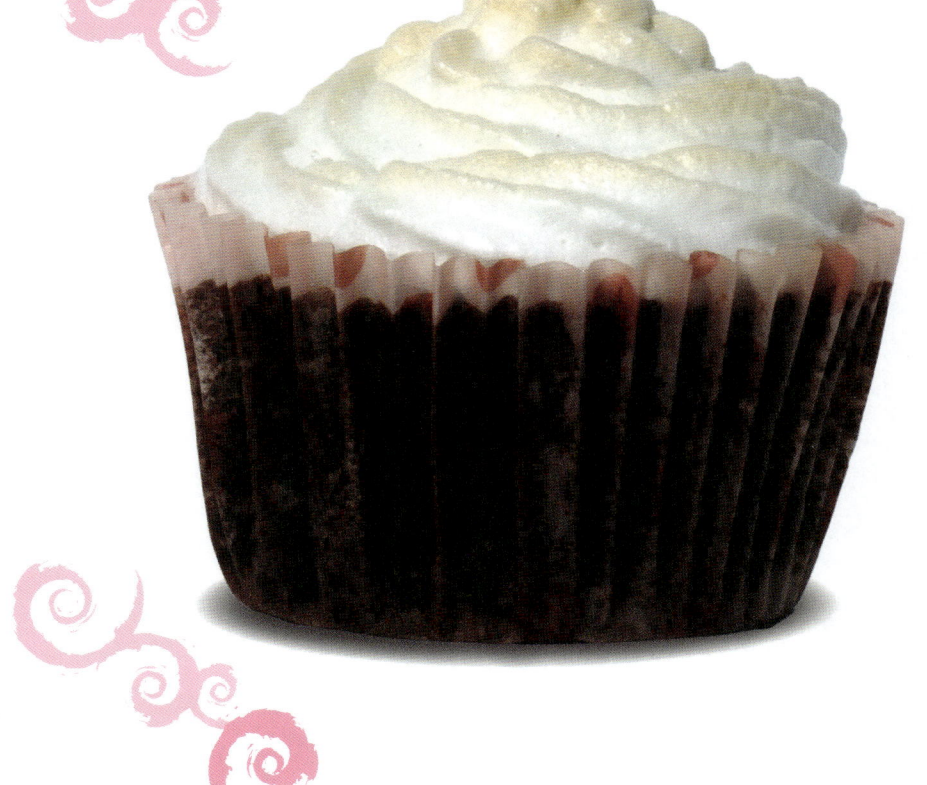

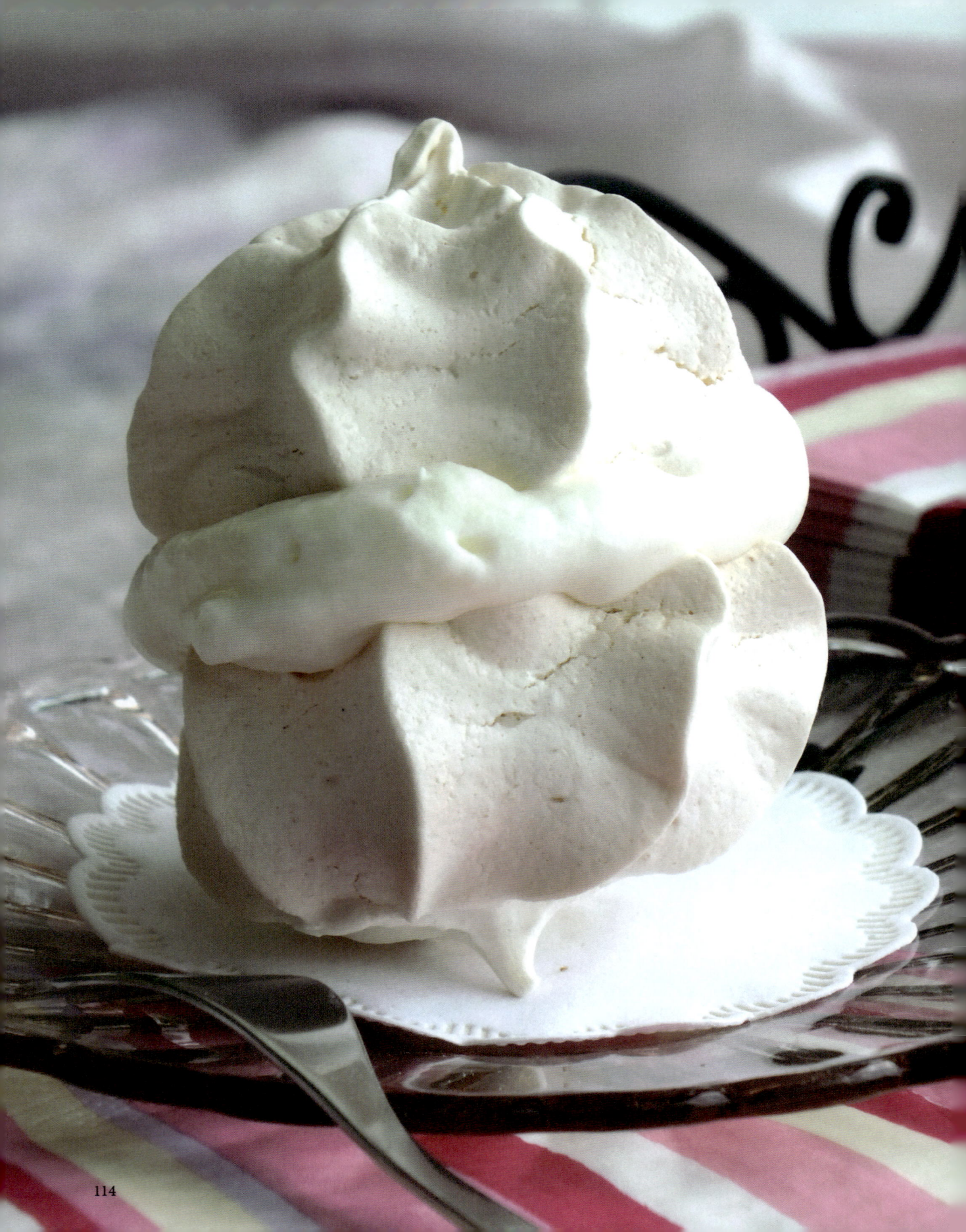

Vanilla Meringue Sandwich Cookies

Yield: 6 extra-large sandwich cookies | Per serving: 1 sandwich cookie – 142 calories

For the cookies:

2 extra-large egg whites, 32 calories

¼ teaspoon fine salt

¾ cup granulated sugar, 150 g, 562 calories

1 teaspoon vanilla extract, 4 g, 12 calories

For the filling:

¼ cup heavy cream (double cream), 60 ml, 200 calories

1 tablespoon granulated sugar, 12 g, 45 calories

¼ teaspoon instant vanilla pudding, 1 g, 3 calories

Cookies:
Preheat the oven to 230°F (110°C).
Line a baking sheet with parchment paper.
Combine egg whites and salt in the bowl of an electric mixer and beat on medium-high speed until soft peaks form. Add the sugar, a little at a time, and continue to beat until the meringue holds very stiff peaks. Beat in the vanilla extract.

Transfer the meringue to a pastry bag fitted with a ½-inch (13 millimeters) star or plain tip. Pipe, equally, twelve cookies in two-inch (five centimeters) rounds on the baking sheet. Alternatively, spoon mounds of meringue, using two spoons, onto the prepared sheets.
Bake for approximately one and a half hours.
The meringues are done when they are fairly crisp.
Turn off the heat and cool the meringues in the oven for an hour, propping the door open with a wooden spoon.

Filling:
Place the heavy cream, sugar, and instant pudding in the bowl of the electric mixer. With the whisk attachment, whip the cream until soft peaks form. Do not overbeat.
Assemble just before serving: take one cookie and spread about 1 tablespoon of the filling on the flat side of the cookie. Top with a second cookie.
The meringue cookies (without the filling) can be stored up to two days at room temperature in airtight containers.

Vanilla Biscotti

Yield: 20 biscotti | Per serving: 2 biscotti – 152 calories; 1 biscotto – 76 calories

1¾ cups all-purpose flour, 228 g, 758 calories

2 teaspoons baking powder

¾ cup granulated sugar, 150 g, 562 calories

¼ teaspoon salt

2 extra-large eggs, 160 calories

1 tablespoon vanilla extract, 13 g, 37 calories

Preheat oven to 350°F (175°C).

Line a baking sheet with parchment paper.

In the bowl of an electric mixer, combine the flour, baking powder, sugar, and salt. In another small bowl, whisk the eggs and vanilla. Gradually add the egg mixture to the flour, and beat until dough forms. If the dough does not form add one to three tablespoons of water.

On a lightly floured surface, roll dough into a log about sixteen inches (forty centimeters) long and two inches (five centimeters) wide. Transfer the log to the prepared baking sheet, and bake for twenty-five to thirty minutes, or until firm to the touch. Let cool for about twenty minutes. Reduce oven temperature to 300°F (150°C).

Transfer log to a cutting board and cut into twenty slices about ½-inch (1¼ cm) thick using a serrated knife. Arrange the slices, cut side down, on the baking sheet. Bake another ten minutes, turn slices over, and bake another ten minutes or until golden brown. Remove from oven and let cool on a wire rack.

Cookies can be stored in an airtight container for a month.

Vanilla Meringue Cookies

Yield: 12 large cookies | Per serving: 2 cookies - 108 calories; 1 cookie - 54 calories

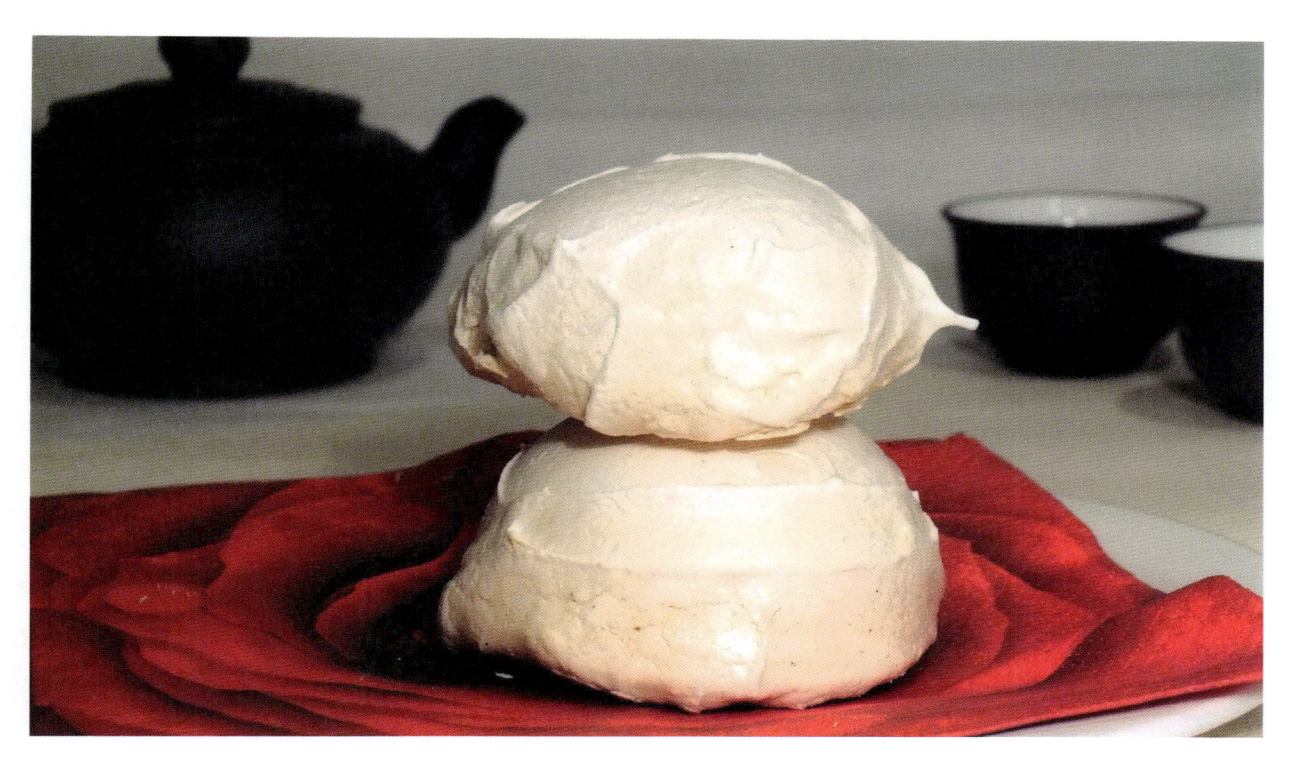

2 extra-large egg whites, 32 calories

¼ teaspoon fine salt

½ teaspoon white vinegar

¾ cup granulated sugar, 150 g, 562 calories

1 tablespoon cornstarch (corn flour), 8 g, 30 calories

1½ teaspoons vanilla extract, 6 g, 18 calories

Preheat oven to 230°F (110°C).
Line a baking sheet with parchment paper.

Combine egg whites, salt, and white vinegar together in the bowl of an electric mixer—the bowl and beaters must be clean and free of grease— and beat on high speed until soft peaks form (about four minutes). Add the sugar, a little at a time, and continue to beat until the meringue holds very stiff peaks. Beat in the vanilla, and then sift in the cornstarch. Use an ice cream scoop or spoon mounds of meringue, using two spoons, onto the prepared sheets. Bake for about two hours, rotating the baking sheet from front to back to ensure even baking. The meringues are done when they are pale in color and fairly crisp.

Turn off the heat and cool the meringues in the oven for an hour, propping the door open with a wooden spoon.
The meringues can be covered and stored up to two days at room temperature in airtight containers.

Vanilla Meringue Chocolate Cupcakes

Yield: 16 cupcakes | Per serving: 1 cupcake – 138 calories

For the cupcakes:

5 tablespoons water

4 ounces semi-sweet chocolate, cut into
½-inch chunks (or ⅔ cup chocolate chips),
112 g, 560 calories

¾ cup all-purpose flour, 98 g, 325 calories

1 tablespoon cocoa powder, 5 g, 10 calories

¾ teaspoon baking powder

¾ teaspoon baking soda

½ cup granulated sugar, 100 g, 375 calories

½ cup unsweetened applesauce, 105 g,
43 calories

¾ cup Greek yogurt 2%, 180 g, 135 calories

1 teaspoon vanilla extract, 4 g, 12 calories

½ cup milk (1% fat), 120 ml, 54 calories

1 extra-large egg, 80 calories

3 extra-large egg yolks, 192 calories

¼ teaspoon fine salt

For the meringue:

2 egg whites at room temperature, 32 calories

¼ teaspoon fine salt

½ cup granulated sugar, 100 g, 375 calories

1 teaspoon vanilla extract, 4 g, 12 calories

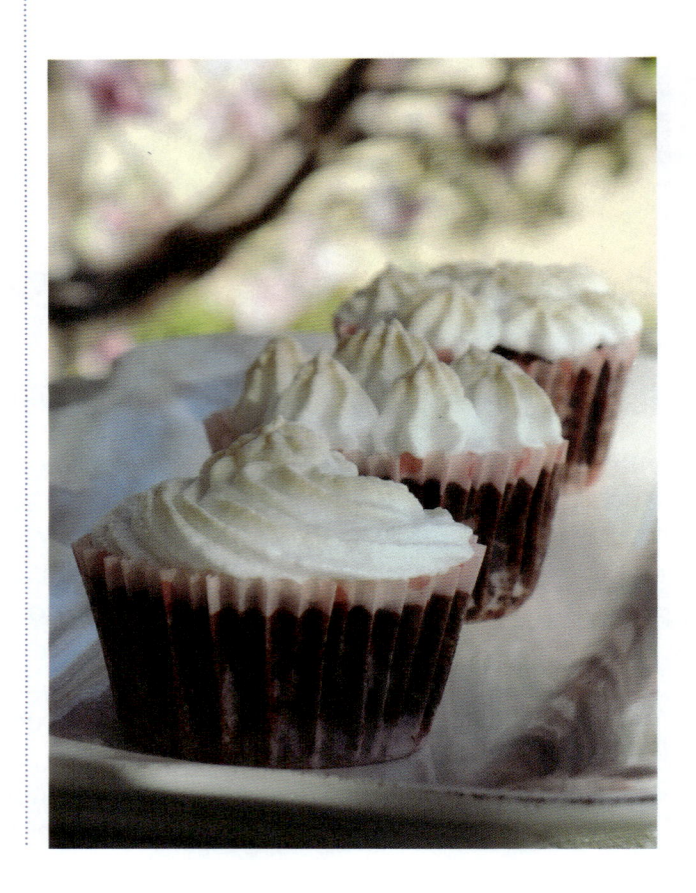

Preheat oven to 340°F (170°C).

Line a standard muffin tin with paper liners (or baking cups) and spray with nonstick baking spray.

Put a pan (or any similar baking dish) with 1 cup of water on the bottom rack of the oven.

Add water to chocolate in a small saucepan over very low heat. Stir until chocolate is melted and mixture is completely smooth. Remove from heat and let cool approximately five minutes.

Sift the flour, cocoa, baking powder, and baking soda together in a large mixing bowl. Mix in the sugar.

Puree the applesauce in a blender or a food processor (the applesauce needs to be finely pureed and smooth) and then measure ½ cup.

In a medium bowl, whisk together the yogurt, vanilla, applesauce, milk, and chocolate mixture. Stir until the mixture is combined and smooth.

With an electric mixer, with the whisk attachment, beat the whole egg, 3 egg yolks, and salt on high speed until the batter is thick and fluffy (about two minutes).

Gently fold the yogurt/chocolate mixture into the eggs until incorporated.

Make a well in the flour mixture, and pour in the liquid mixture. Stir just to combine (don't over-mix or you will have tough cupcakes).

Use an ice cream scoop to distribute the batter evenly among the baking cups, filling each 80 percent full. Bake for approximately twenty to twenty-five minutes until firm but not fully baked.

Make the meringue when the cupcakes are in the oven. With an electric mixer—the bowl and beaters must be clean and free of grease—beat the egg whites on medium-high speed until foamy. Add the salt and continue to beat until they hold soft peaks. Add the sugar, a little at a time, and continue to beat until the meringue holds very stiff peaks. Beat in the vanilla extract until combined. Transfer meringue to a pastry bag fitted with a small open-star tip.

Remove the cupcakes from the oven, and pipe five to seven starbursts around the perimeter of the warm cupcakes, then pipe another starburst in the center. Return to the oven and bake about five minutes. Do not over-bake or you will have dry cupcakes.

Cool in the pan for a few minutes before removing to a cooling rack.

Cupcakes can be refrigerated up to two days in airtight containers. Bring to room temperature before serving.

Index

Notes

Notes

Notes

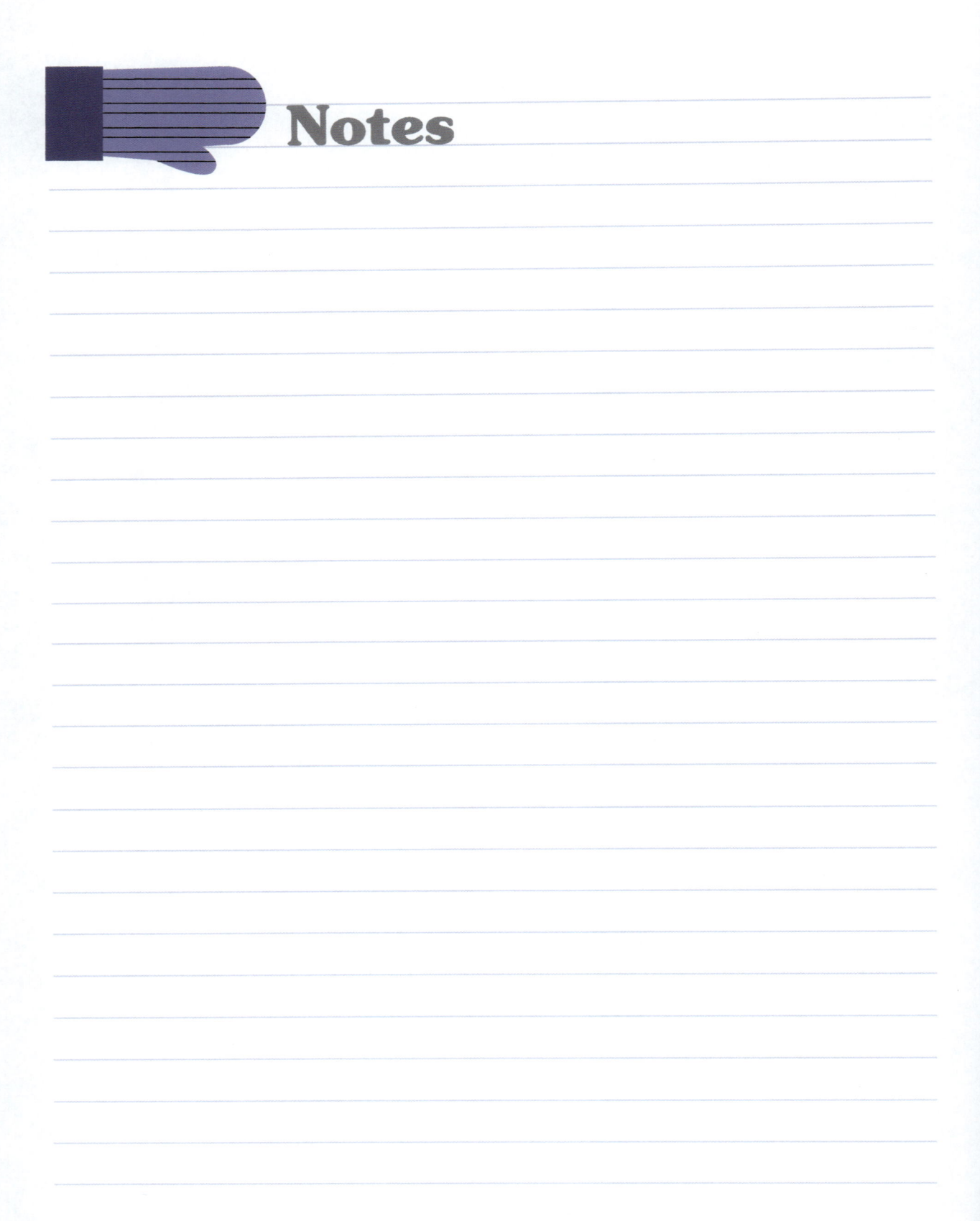

2433078R00065

Printed in Great Britain
by Amazon.co.uk, Ltd.,
Marston Gate.